REFLECTIONS

A CARETAKER'S BATTLE WITH ALZHEIMER'S DISEASE

Donna M. Hayes

ISBN: 1500978108
ISBN 13: 9781500978105
Library of Congress Control Number: 2014915662
CreateSpace Independent Publishing Platform
North Charleston, South Carolina

DEDICATED TO THE CARETAKER

In loving memory of my mother, Corinne,
Forever I am changed by your love.

TABLE OF CONTENTS

PREFACE

L ife can sometimes break you open, reach into your soul, and unearth your emotional roots when you least expect it and are least prepared for it. This is what happened to me when my mother's life collided with Alzheimer's disease, a form of dementia.

There are pamphlets, books, and countless Internet sites about the science of Alzheimer's disease, and the care needed for your loved one. This is not a book about the disease itself or the particulars of what this disease did to my mother. It is a book about how I coped and did not cope. It is written for the person who is on the front lines of this disease – the caretaker.

Initially, Alzheimer's assault was slow and subtle affecting my mother marginally causing nominal demands and disturbance on my life. However, as her disease gained momentum, it not only attacked my mother but also my physical and mental health. Facing foreign situations, decisions, and emotions with diminished energy and clarity further depleted my wellbeing, and created turmoil in my marriage.

Retrospectively, I wished that someone had told me of the diverse struggles I would inevitably face but that victory was possible. After my mother died, I was compelled to revisit my journals to share my innermost thoughts with future caretakers. It is from this place that I offer you hope. I wrote this book for all those people who, unknowingly, belong to a secret society whose members' lives intersect with Alzheimer's disease.

I realized I was part of this secret society while shopping with my mother for a birthday card. Standing behind Mom's wheelchair in the card aisle, I read her card after card, hoping to share a laugh and select our favorite to send to my brother. A woman around fifteen years older than me stood eight feet to our left, also reading cards. Something as uncomplicated and fun as selecting a card became a difficult chore. As Mom battled my every word, the woman interrupted her search, glanced in our direction, intentionally replaced her card to the stack, and began walking toward us. She stopped by my side, dropped her head, put her left hand on my left shoulder, and held it there for several seconds. I said nothing, and she said nothing. Her deafening silence and defeated posture conveyed a journey that wounded her so profoundly that it transcended words. In my silence I understood that she had been where I now was. She had finished what I had just begun. She knew my life without knowing me at all. She was not passing me a baton to finish running a victorious race; she was passing me a baton, hoping in empathy that my fate would somehow be different. I wanted to fall at her feet and beg desperately for answers. What is my fate? What was your experience? What did you learn? How did it affect your marriage? However, the woman did not allow me access into the archives of her mind. Instead, with a heavy hand she patted my shoulder and walked away out of my invisible, desperate grip.

Her gesture, so brave, so intimate, made me realize that I was not alone but part of the secret society of Alzheimer's caretakers. A society you did not know you joined but became a lifetime member of. A society where knowing the other members was not a requirement. A society whose dues would cost us all dearly.

JANUARY 2004–
JANUARY 2006

DEFINING AND MEETING THE ENEMY

"Corinne, can I see you climb the steps?" Mom, a widow of six years, insisted on living alone in Philadelphia. Every eight weeks I traveled to Philadelphia from Houston for three weeks to care for her. Initially my concern was for her physical safety while climbing the steep steps of her four-story three-thousand-square-foot row house. Knee pain forced Mom to climb the staircase on all fours. When I visited I'd propel Mom upward with my hands placed on her behind. In the morning my hands cupped her underarms while she gripped the banister sideways one step at a time, but inevitably knee pain forced her to end the descent on her butt.

To validate my concern that she should not be living alone, I invited a geriatric nurse to evaluate Mom and the safety of her home. If either failed the test, I would have a professional's opinion endorsing my position. Mom, like a veteran soldier, marched toward her duty station, halting at the base of the steps. Standing at attention, she placed her left hand firmly on the banister and began her ascent straight-backed without flinching. I knew her knees were on fire with pain. When she was halfway up, the nurse applauded Mom and passed her with an approving smile. Mom marched down the steps with the same cadence. I shot her an accusatory look: "You actress!" "You phony!" Her responding smile told me that she outsmarted me once again. However, as my visits continued, Mom's physical condition became secondary to her mental state.

One morning my brother, Mario, and I received a frantic call from Mom after she received a letter from the hospital reporting a diagnosis of Alzheimer's disease. A few weeks prior she had fallen, hit her head on the cement sidewalk, and admitted herself to the emergency room, where they, unknown to us, did a brain scan. These were the results. We had been monitoring changes in Mom's unusual behavior but, in our denial, attributed them to her age of seventy-five. In light of this new information, we began researching this disease, linking its symptoms to her strange behavior.

Mom had become suspicious over the past year. Trusting her memory so completely when things were not where she remembered them to be, she concluded that people were stealing from her. To catch the thieves she began writing her name on every grocery item in the house and hiding them and everything of value in the most bizarre places. During one of my visits, I put a load of laundry in the washer and went out with a friend. On the ride home I asked Elaine to borrow her cell phone to call Mom.

"Hello."

"Hi, Mom, it's me. The clothes should be done. But before you put them into the dryer, remove the cans of tomato sauce."

"I already did."

"Great. I'll see you in a bit."

After hanging up, I looked over at Elaine, who was grinning from ear to ear. I said, "You realize I couldn't have had that conversation in front of too many people." "Donna, I understand...you know I understand."

Elaine's mother, eighty-nine, also lived alone in another state, with signs of dementia. We had shared many stories about our mothers' strange behavior and our failed attempts at long-distance damage control.

In trying to honor Mom's wishes to live alone, we made necessary adjustments for her daily needs. My brother stayed with her on weekends and filled her weekly pillbox. From Houston, my job was to call Mom twice daily to instruct her to take her medications. One day after church my husband, Paul, wanted to stop at a golf shop.

"I'll be in. I have to call Mom to take her medication."

A once-simple task of calling Mom became an exhausting two-hour daily chore. Many times I would call, and she would lay the phone down in the dining room and go into the kitchen to take her pills. While searching for the pillbox, she would forget the phone was off the hook. I would then call the neighbors, and they would ring the bell to tell her to put the phone back on the hook so I could call again to make sure she took her pills. This morning, however, we did not go through this frustrating and tedious ritual.

"Hi, Mom, it's time to take your medicine."

"Don't 'hi, Mom' me! I'm so disappointed in you."

"What did I do?"

"You know what you did!"

"No, I don't. What did I do?"

"You stole my jewelry!"

I was stunned yet perplexed. Logic pled my defense.

"You're telling me that I flew to Philadelphia last night from Houston, took a cab from the airport, told him to wait for me, snuck into the house, stole your jewelry, drove back to the airport, and flew back to Houston in time to call you?"

"That's exactly what I'm saying."

I froze, unable to speak or scarcely breathe. This was not just old age. No. This was something bigger. Something that stood unashamed, defying logic while holding the mother I knew hostage. This was my first encounter with the enemy: Alzheimer's.

JANUARY 2007– JANUARY 2009

SPARRING WITH THE ENEMY

When I first got married in 1998, I quit my job because my husband's work relocated us overseas for six and a half years. Then in 2004 his job relocated us back to the States to Houston, Texas. After settling into our new home, I thought about working again, but caring for Mom long distance along with my frequent trips to Philadelphia became a full-time job. In 2007 my husband retired, but they rehired him for an assignment in Rome, Italy, starting immediately. We had lived overseas before, but this relocation escalated the anxiety and tension I felt between being a wife and a caretaking daughter. We put our Houston home up for sale, hoping to relocate closer to Mom in Philadelphia upon our return. We packed our computer and a few suitcases and left. My visits to Mom continued from Italy but were less frequent due to cost. To manage Mom and the taking of her daily medications, I arranged for a special overseas phone line and set up speed dial, taping a list of family and neighbors by her phone.

Because I lived in another country, and my brother lived an hour and a half away from Mom, Mario and I formed a plan to manage her long distance. He would stay with her on Sundays and Mondays, and we hired a woman to stay from Tuesdays to Saturdays from 9:00 a.m. to 6:00 p.m. Maggie's duties were to take my mother food shopping, clean the house, and, most importantly, make sure Mom ate. Not understanding the time difference, Mom would call me at 6:00 p.m., not knowing it was 2:00 a.m. in Europe, to scream to me about Maggie: "This woman is still in my house! I don't want her cleaning my kitchen."

I would then call my brother, who advised me not to answer the phone, hoping they would work it out and become friendly companions. It killed me not to answer the phone as it rang night after night. Two weeks later Maggie called me; Mom had locked her out of the house. We needed a new plan. In the meantime my brother began staying with Mom seven days a week, extending his already long job commute.

I tried living my life, but thoughts of Mom's welfare continually distracted me throughout my day, especially when food shopping, which was one of Mom's favorite activities. Unlike the Italian women who food shopped daily, I would shop at the outdoor food market a few times a week. Every time I was there, a tall, strong-looking Italian woman caught my eye. Gripping her arm was her short, thin, feeble, partially blind mother, who captured my heart. Transfixed by the reversal in role and stature, I would stop, inundated with compassion by the daughter's strength and patience, eclipsed only by the mother's humility. Envying that she had her mother with her, I wondered what her daily life was like. As I watched them disappear into the crowd, shopping became inconsequential as my eyes continually searched for this poignant duo, and my heart ached to know that Mom was safe. I wondered if anyone else saw them through empathetic eyes the way I did. No one else seemed to. People only became exasperated trying to navigate around these two women and their toddler pace.

My brother, always looking for ways for Mom to live a full life in spite of Alzheimer's, decided to take her and my niece to visit us in Italy. The night before they were to leave, I received a phone call that Mom hid her passport, resulting in a frantic search. Mario and his daughter, Julia, searched every one of Mom's known hiding places from past scavenger hunts but found it nowhere. After three hours of intense searching, they discovered it in a new hiding place: inside the cuckoo clock. Of course. Where else would you keep your passport?

Since Mom's house was next to a Sicilian bakery with the best cannoli ever, my husband asked if she would bring him some. Mom, always the dutiful servant, especially to her son-in-law, held the cannoli in a death grip into the cab, on the plane, and into the airplane's bathroom, not trusting their care to anyone. There were no issues on the plane except that after the movie Mom wanted to leave, believing they were at the movie theater. Mom's reality was unique and insulated, having little relationship with what was going on around her. She lived in a world of her own and just followed my brother's lead.

They arrived safely at my front door by early afternoon along with the cannoli. With much of the day ahead of them, my brother and niece decided to visit the Vatican, while Mom rested and spent time with me. As they began heading down the steps to the front door, Mom, knowing Mario was her way home to Philadelphia, began running toward him, screaming, "Don't leave me here! Don't leave me here!"

I had to restrain her physically so they could leave. Her violent response evidenced the enemy's continued advance. Calming her down came only by guaranteeing their return by proof of their luggage.

Their visit went well even though Mom had no idea where she was. Location, at this stage in her life, was unimportant to her. What was important was that she was with family. Family was paramount to my mother. Two weeks of touring and eating ended, and they returned home to Philadelphia, where Mom was most comfortable.

After fourteen months in Italy, my husband retired a second time. We returned to our home in Houston, which, regretfully, had not sold. I reluctantly reestablished my residence, delaying my hope to live closer to Mom. I took every precaution I could think of for her safety. For example, I made ten different lanyards with the house key hanging off the end. She wore one around her neck. I hid the other nine around the house before I left for Houston, anticipating that she would lose the one around her neck. When she did, I instructed her over the phone to the hidden location of one of the other nine lanyards. One morning at six I received a phone call from Mom's neighbor. Since time was relative to being awake, and the lines between morning and night were blurred, Mom, ready for church, walked out of the house at 4:00 a.m. believing it was 4:00 p.m. Forgetting to wear the lanyard around her neck, she had locked herself out of the house. The baker next door, who began his day at 4:00 a.m., took her in. Other times neighbors would tell me she would knock on their doors looking for her mother as the enemy, Alzheimer's, tricked her into thinking her mother was still alive.

On another morning my brother called at five-thirty, informing me that he just received a call from the police, who had picked Mom up and escorted her home. Mom's disposition changed from quiet to aggressive in her disease. This particular event happened because she was convinced that her closest sister, Gloria, had stolen her cinnamon buns. Therefore, at 3:00 a.m., my enraged mother walked two city blocks to her sister's house and began pounding on her front door and screaming that she give up the cinnamon buns. Her sister, frightened, called the police. I did not have a juvenile delinquent. I had a senior delinquent.

Mom also began letting strangers into the house. During one of my brother's evening calls, she told him of the nice man Mitch and his wife who she was entertaining. My brother, believing she was hallucinating because she continually saw little children in the house, asked to speak to Mitch to verify his belief. When Mitch got on the phone, my brother became alarmed and demanded to know who he was and why he was in his mother's house. They were the new neighbors who bought Mom's sister's house after she died—the sister who headed up the cinnamon-bun caper. They found Mom at their door looking for her sister and brought her home. On my next visit I stopped by to see Mitch and his wife, only to discover that they, too, belonged to the secret society, thereby understanding her confusion.

Having a type-A personality, I like to be in control of my life. However, as Mom's emotional state declined and her need for daily monitoring increased, I began to experience a low level of panic. My efficient, organized, and controlled life was becoming progressively difficult to maintain. My trips to Philadelphia went from every eight weeks for three weeks to every six weeks for three weeks. Whenever I arrived back in Houston, before I knew it, it was time to leave again for Philadelphia. To stay in control I only left my home in Houston after cleaning, doing the laundry, paying the bills, and cooking to stock the freezer with enough food for my husband during my absence. Once I arrived in Philadelphia, I would do the same for my mother. Every visit presented new logistical challenges not only to my own life but, more importantly, to ensure Mom's safety for the upcoming weeks. Whatever city I was in I continued exploring new medical advances against the enemy, Alzheimer's. My favorite place of solace was at the airport in between destinations, where I had no role to fill but one—that of a stranger. It was a role I gladly embraced. There I would hope and pray for a flight delay because no one knew where I was or needed me. However, always lurking in the back of my mind was how I was losing every battle against the enemy.

RECONNAISSANCE ON THE ENEMY

There are rules defining the conduct of a just war, identifying how it should and should not be fought, weapons considered evil, and combatants from noncombatant civilians. Alzheimer's, being an unethical and merciless terrorist, ignores all conduct of war, just or otherwise, with one aim: to destroy. His targets are soft, taking mostly elderly civilians hostage, exploiting them while victimizing other noncombatants: their families. His military maneuvers are all encompassing, causing daily interruptions, economic destruction, social disruption, and emotional eruptions.

Even the terrain of this war is different from any other. It is not hills versus flat ground. It is not a battle of wits, manpower, or weaponry. It is not a traditional or primitive war but a highly complex and unconventional one fought in an invisible arena.

The enemy was a mole. His basecamp was in my mother's mind; therefore, he knew my intelligence and defeated my every move. Regardless of how many times I tried to act, the enemy's offensive posture always forced me into a weak defensive position: one of reaction. There were two campaigns underway, one against my mother and one against me. His tactics were extremely effective because every time he launched an attack against Mom, he struck me. We were one, connected by love.

WEAPONOLOGY

The enemy's weapons were not conventional but futuristic. They were biomolecular, making his attacks invisible to the naked eye and perceived only after the damage was assessed. The consequences of his weaponry caused biological, psychological, and chemical ramifications for my mother. Mario and I endlessly investigated every possible weapon to fight this unusual enemy, but it's difficult to forge weapons after the war begins. Our findings directed us into trying every natural remedy with promise while putting her on every drug study available from the hospital—drug studies that demanded countless MRIs, which, for an Alzheimer's patient, was next to impossible. Antianxiety drugs did not keep her still during the MRI. Therefore, I would accompany Mom into the MRI room, ending up with half my body literally inside the machine, trying to hold her still. MRI days were extremely difficult days for both of us.

In addition to all the drug studies, my brother and I decided to meet with a staff of eight from a special neurology unit in the hospital to see if they could offer any additional help. At our meeting we shared stories of Mom's strange behavior that they had all heard before. They instructed me to leave her the next day for two nights of observation at the hospital.

The next morning Mom and I walked to the hospital in the city center. The elevator doors opened to an austere hallway on an upper floor. I immediately knew this was a special floor—a floor where one was not invited but summoned by desperation. The environment was chilling and void of color, rugs, or a warm welcome. I pressed the hand-sized, round, stainless-steel buzzer that sent shockwaves down my spine. As they unlocked the two large glass doors, the sounds, with piercing clarity, echoed off the cold surfaces. The doors opened to another benign, sterile environment that provided no comfort or color except for one small TV surrounded by elderly, seemingly forgotten women. They showed me the room where my mother would sleep for her two-day stay in these haunting accommodations; there was a chair and a cold metal bed with a strap connected to a bed alarm to prevent night wanderings. Part of their welcoming protocol was testing the deafening, Nazi-like siren, which transported horror into the depth of one's soul.

Unsuccessfully, I tried to ease Mom into the other women's company, but she separated herself. I left reluctantly, hoping their observations would provide some answers. That night sleep evaded me as thoughts of Mom tossed and turned in my mind. After the first day I took her out to K-mart since it was across from the hospital—anything to get her out of that environment. On the second morning I sprinted to the hospital, breathlessly entering the slow-moving elevator. Like a lioness, I paced its small perimeter, questioning why it took so long to go four floors. The elevator stopped. My heart was pounding as another four protracted seconds passed. Finally the doors began to open. I forced my body through the slowly appearing crack. They buzzed me in, but I did not see my mother with the other women surrounding the small TV. I asked the attendant, "Where is she?"

"She's in her room."

She was not in her room. Frantically, I ran from room to room like a mother who temporarily lost her child in a crowded park. While running down the hallway at a frenzied pace, I bumped into Mom calmly walking out of someone else's room, unaware of my distress, with a *Reader's Digest* in hand. She loved this magazine but now looked more at the pictures and was only able to read the highlighted boxes. I hugged her forcefully, spinning her around and checking for damage like a mother who had located her wandering child. While I was questioning myself as to the profit of all this, an attendant opened a locked-down area where screams emerged from patients who had lost their minds. The thought of her ending up in a place like this overwhelmed me. I had to get her out of there as soon as possible. I told them to discharge her without any observation results, and we left.

On the walk home I condemned myself for having to rescue her from a situation that we created and began my internal chastising interrogation. *How could I have left her there? What were we thinking? Why did we even make that decision? Was it the neurologist's suggestion?* I could not remember. Desperation was the only answer. I looked over at Mom as we walked. She did not remember anything about the past two days. With the innocence of a child, she just held my hand, trusting I was leading her to a safe place. My heart continued to break into pieces, knowing that any success was temporary as this enemy called Alzheimer's annihilated every defensive measure I tried. With every step I took, my mind raced, desperately seeking new strategies to prevent the enemy from gaining more ground.

My three weeks in my role as caretaking daughter ended, and I returned to Houston to fill my role as wife. Leaving her alone with the enemy was torture for me. From a torn heart I would pray for God's hand of protection over her. When I arrived back in Houston, I once again hit the ground running: shopping, cooking, unpacking, cleaning, doing laundry, budgeting, and paying bills while managing Mom and the enemy at a distance.

FEBRUARY 2009–MARCH 2009

KIDNAPPED

Another three weeks passed, and I had planned to visit Mom in three more weeks but received an urgent call from my brother. Our mother had burned herself badly, and he found a charred dishtowel hidden in the kitchen drawer. He firmly felt that she could not be left alone, fearing she might burn down the house. I left immediately, unaware that it would be my last trip like this from Houston.

When I opened the front door, I found Mom's row home dark and quiet. "Mom? Mom!" Hearing no response, I stood at the base of the steps listening to her talking to herself and other imaginary friends while going through drawers ad nauseam—her constant daily activity. Leaning against the banister to the second floor, I could only cry, assessing the woman she once was and the woman she had become since her capture.

My mother was always a quiet, soft, reserved, patient, gentle, inquisitive, giving, humble, and smart woman. She was able to think outside the box, had great ideas, and always wanted to do the right thing. At her core she was a traditional woman. Although I respected and embraced her traditions, I did not like the parts that restricted individual expression and independence. At our essence Mom and I were completely different people. I was outspoken, aggressive, artistic, inpatient, and, as a teenager, always looking for the loophole to get away from doing the right thing. I always believed she would have rather had my cousin Marlene as her daughter. Marlene was very much like my Mom, unlike me, who always locked horns with my mother. Mom did not understand me, nor did she try, resting on the fact that she was the mother and I was the daughter. The unspoken mandate was for me to assume my role and never challenge her in any way. We loved one another, but we did not like one another. We tolerated each other. In my heart I wished I had been the daughter she hoped for, but I knew that ever since I was a child, in her eyes I fell short at my assigned role and her expectations of me. This, however, was not the time to ponder my feelings. The truth lay before me. We were two different people on the same side fighting one unseen enemy.

Putting our contrasting relationship aside, I climbed the steep steps to the second floor. She was elated to see me, but I was shocked to see how much weight she had lost in just three weeks and how disheveled she looked in forgetting to shower or eat. Later that day after returning from the food store, I found Mom lying on the floor. At eighty years old, Mom had decided to stand on a chair to clean the kitchen ceiling, lost her balance, and fell onto her feeble knees. Now she was unable to walk, and my brother carried her up seventeen steps to bed and then down again in the morning. He carried her in and out of cabs, into the doctor's office and out of the doctor's office. We were both exhausted, and my three-week trip turned into five weeks. Her knees, void of cartilage, were slow in healing, making it impossible for me to leave.

My husband called, asking when I was coming home. I did not have an answer to his question nor the question that plagued me constantly: How can I be a good wife and a good, caretaking daughter at the same time? He suggested that she come and live with us in our one-story Houston home. However, Mom ignored this suggestion made many times to her in the past. Mom always said she did not want to burden her children, adding a guilt-laced caveat that "loving children do not put their parents 'away.'" She had taken care of her parents, her older brother, my father, and the two of us. These were her seeds sown and the harvest she expected to reap. She was not to come to us; we were to come to her home and care for her there. Mom never lived anywhere else. This was where she grew up, where she lived her married life, and where she raised my brother and me. A stubborn and strong-willed Sicilian woman, she was living the rest of her years right there, and we could not pry her out of the sanctuary she called home.

This home is where her immigrant parents began their marriage and where they raised their eight children. It had been in the family for 109 years, becoming a refuge to her seven siblings even though they now had homes of their own, except for Mom. Since she cared for her elderly father, she inherited the house and remained there. No one referred to it as the family house or Mom's house or their parents' house, or Corinne's house—just "1011" and, in so doing, christened the address as its name. Mom loved 1011 so much that it became personified as her second son. Severing the umbilical cord was next to impossible.

My mind raced for a solution to move Mom out of the house but to no avail. I concluded that I had to think unorthodox thoughts that in normal circumstances I would never entertain. With apprehension, I called my brother and suggested that we kidnap her. Surprisingly, he agreed. The night before, sadness and guilt engulfed me, knowing this would be her last night in her home of eighty years. With the premeditation of a criminal, I showered Mom and put her to bed in her street clothes. At 2:00 a.m. I gave her a powerful sedative. At 3:30 a.m. my brother called a cab then carried her down the steps and into the cab. In retrospect I could only imagine what the cabdriver thought, but, in the moment, we were criminals functioning like clockwork according to our devious plan—all for Mom's safety. We arrived at the airport for a five-thirty flight to Houston with a doctor's note explaining Mom's condition in case authorities questioned our motives. Mario carried our drugged mother to her first-class seat among a sea of onlookers. It was the worst night of my life. After the plane took off, I looked back at my brother for reassurance that we were doing the right thing, but he was fast asleep. A drugged Mom rested by my side while I sat wide awake, paralyzed by self-contempt. After a few hours breakfast arrived, and I began trying to feed my groggy, barely coherent mother. One of the flight attendants commented on how good I was with Mom. Even though I was fifty years old, I felt like a disobedient daughter doing something my mother would not condone. I was going against her every desire, strong arming her without her knowledge—another example to myself why I felt I was not a good daughter in her eyes and one she did not like. I just smiled back at the flight attendant, unable to receive her intended compliment.

My husband met us on the other end with a wheel-chair. He was happy for the move because it meant that I would not be gone every six weeks for three weeks. We arrived home, which he furnished with the necessary equipment specific for her elderly needs. My brother stayed the weekend and left for the airport on Monday morning. When she awoke, she forgot that my brother had been there. Our plan worked, and she thought she was in Philadelphia. We tricked her, and I felt horrible. I was the daughter who was not loyal to the one person in my life who had been most loyal to me. It was March 9, 2009. Mom was eighty, and for the next three years my life, my heart, and my soul would be changed forever.

MARCH 9, 2009–
DECEMBER 31, 2009

LIVING WITH THE ENEMY

Beside my bed in Houston rested a baby monitor. Its green glistening light was under my constant surveillance as I was anticipating that Mom would need bathroom care. Every bed rustle or sleep-talking sound sent me running down the long hallway that separated her room from ours. Eventually I just began sleeping in the single bed next to hers. In the ten months she lived with us, she was never out of my sight except on the rare occasion when she was with my husband.

Over the next few weeks, her knees healed, and she was again mobile. She was okay walking on a flat surface for a short time while holding on to furniture here and there; however, I mostly kept her in the transport chair because she preferred it.

Before the disease Mom was a great cook. Now she sat in my kitchen while I cooked for her, increasing her weight to 110 pounds, which she desperately needed. I cut her hair into a new style, gave her a new hair color, and bought her new clothes and new eyeglasses. Being a homemaker did not afford Mom the luxury of painting her nails. Therefore, one day I took her shopping to pick out nail polish. To my surprise Mom picked hot pink. It was so unlike the pale colors she would wear to an occasional wedding. Now she would sit and enjoy her manicures. Throughout the day I would see her extending her hand, viewing her nails in admiration. In these moments I would delude myself by thinking that everything was going great. I was able to exhale, believing Mom and I would begin building our relationship on a different foundation. When I told her it was "beauty day," she would laugh with excitement. For a woman who was almost eighty-one, she now looked seventy-one.

My brother began visiting every few months. His first visit was in May to celebrate Mother's Day and Mom's eighty-first birthday. When he walked in and Mom saw him, she first jumped out of her skin with joy then jumped out of her chair to get to him. I cried to see her so happy while at the same time wishing she were that happy to be with me. Knowing how I made Mom look ten years younger and wanting Mario's approval that I was taking good care of her, I proudly asked, "How does Mom look?"

"She looks great, but you look terrible."

I didn't care what I looked like. I just wanted Mom to be fine because when she was fine, my heart was fine. While I was searching for a response to his comment, my bizarre daily existence flashed before me.

The truth was that I lost the weight she gained and was holding at ninety-seven pounds. I looked terrible because my body functioned on autopilot. I had not slept at night for more than twenty minutes here and there. Normal sleep was literally not a part of my life anymore.

When I finally did get to see a doctor a year later, he said my system had been running like a car in neutral with the gas pedal pushed down to the floor while someone endlessly poured oil into the engine. Racing inside, night after night, I lay in the bed next to Mom with my eyes wide open. Like a readied soldier, I slept in street clothes, never knowing when outside duty would call. Every night Mom awoke either wanting to make meatballs or to go back home, not knowing home was over a thousand miles away. Other nights she was just combative, demanding I open the front door so she could walk home. To keep her calm I opened the front door to her freedom. Victoriously, she would leave, stopped only by the darkness of the driveway. Spinning around with tears rolling down her cheeks, she would plead with me in a quivering voice replete with frustration, "Why are you doing this to me?" Never having an answer, I would just look down at the ground blurred by tears of compassion. I had never seen my mother cry until then, and she believed I was the catalyst, but I was not the guilty one—it was the enemy.

On another night at 2:30 a.m., at the end of the long hallway that separated the two bedrooms, she was ornery and talking loudly. Not wanting to wake my husband, I asked her to keep her voice down. When she refused, I covered her mouth with my hand. She—no, the enemy inside her—went ballistic and began swinging at me, wrapping her hands around my neck and ripping off my necklace. Shocked by her violent behavior, I clutched my neck for damage, but her actions did not faze her in the least; the enraged enemy inside her kept coming at me in hand-to-hand combat. For a four-foot-eight woman, Mom was strong and the enemy within hostile and aggressive. While trying to restrain Mom without hurting her, I thought that if I did have to put her in a memory-care center, I was happy that she knew how to defend herself if someone crossed her boundaries. By 4:00 a.m., she ran out of fight and fell asleep. These were the hours when I would try to care for myself.

Some mornings I went to the gym at 4:00 a.m. On other mornings I set her breakfast table, prepared her coffee pot to decrease my husband's workload, and left at 6:00 a.m. to arrive at seven for therapy to ease my hip pain from a sports injury; this acute pain plagued me daily now, exacerbated by tending to Mom. My treatment ended at 8:00 a.m., and I raced home by nine to relieve my husband from breakfast duty.

When Mom was well, my husband and she got along famously, but now he resented her and the entire situation—especially that he was not receiving my undivided attention as he had for the past eleven years. Now he had to share me with Mom. After the first two months of caring for Mom, my husband, seeing how it was depleting me, suggested I put her into a home. Although his advice was logical, his equation did not take into account the emotional component—my emotions, to be specific. I was not emotionally ready for such a decision; therefore, I did not make it. I had to know beyond any doubt that I tried my best to care for Mom as she had for her parents. I was happy that she lived with me because I did not have any worry about her safety. Because I did not heed my husband's advice, he carved a life out for himself for the ten months Mom lived with us and supported me only when asked or minimally when offered. I knew 10:00

a.m. was his tee time to golf all day and that he would not return until dinner.

Whenever he was home, the atmosphere was tense. Mom felt it, and I knew it. With one hand I was caring for Mom, and with the other I managed his anger. He hated when she swung at me or spoke nastily to me. I tried explaining to him that it was the disease, not her. Over time I learned how to separate the person from the disease. Otherwise the disease wins, and you become filled with hate, victimizing the person more than the enemy already did. Alzheimer's is ruthless, and its diverse arsenal blindsides you: explosive mood swings, inappropriate behavior, and Alzheimer's favorite ploy: pitting people against one another. My husband did not understand, nor did I at the time, that the enemy, in the process of attacking Mom, had a secondary mission: to annihilate our marriage by starting a civil war.

Not to fuel his anger further, I quickly pulled into the garage from my seven-o'clock therapy session and raced into the kitchen, only to see Mom's rigid and fearful posture change to one of relief. While bending down to kiss her, she grabbed my face and whispered, "He's nasty." He had crossed my line—the one I drew in front of my mother. However, because I lacked energy and fight, the angry force surging inside me diminished into extreme disappointment. The one person who professed love for me did not love the one whom I loved the most and taught me how to love him. His attitude not only added to my high stress levels but also demanded that I intensify my efforts, already on life support. I immediately relieved him of breakfast duty while reflecting on all meals my mother and I graciously cooked for him and his three children over the past eleven years. In those minutes every fiber of my being adjudicated that my marriage would become a casualty of this war before my need to care for and honor Mom. Caring for her was so deeply primal to my heart and soul that nothing and no one was going to stand in my way or give me cause to live with regret. He did not understand that when he was loving toward her, he was loving toward me. And when he was nasty to her, in essence he was being nasty to me. That morning my heart began shutting down, and I lost all security, wondering if in any future-case scenario I would be emotionally abandoned again. When he finally left for golf, the atmosphere decompressed, and we both exhaled.

Mornings were unpredictable. Sometimes they went great, and other days it took me until 1:00 p.m. to get her into the shower or dressed. On other mornings after breakfast, Mom would walk out the door to go home. Any attempt at getting her back into the house resulted in a shouting match in the driveway for commuting neighbors to see. On one such occasion the new neighbors that moved in across the street, whom I had all intentions to meet and greet with a welcoming gift, watched, wondering if they had made the right move.

Because I would not take her home, Mom, donning her nightgown and with an angry, defiant stomp, would blaze a trail to Philadelphia from Houston. Knowing her volatility, I followed at a safe distance, hiding behind the large, brick, suburban mailboxes as if I were playing hide and go seek with my mother. The street was always abuzz with the sound of yardmen's tools. I wondered how ridiculous I must have looked to the groups of yardmen working on the manicured lawns. Being a city girl, I felt invaded by these men and the constant buzzing sound from their trimming machines. Nevertheless, I was a daily fixture in their mornings as they were in mine. After seeing them many mornings, I would wave as if we were acquainted, but they would just stop, turn off their machines, and watch in confusion as my daily drama unfolded. Most of these men could not speak English well, but their countenances told me they did not know whether I was abusing the woman and if they should call the cops or if I was helping her. Over time I did not care because I had a different reality than most people. Daily life became a series of crises, and this was just the first one of the day.

The combination of Houston's oppressive heat and her knee pain curtailed Mom's journey. While reaching down to massage her knees, she would look around for help. I cautiously approached her to provide comfort, but with tear-filled frustration she would scream her daily question, "Why are you doing this to me?" I just stood there with my head dropped, tears thwarting my speech. I never knew what to say anyway, but I knew her thought: I was a bad daughter. Nevertheless, I knew this was tough love. With minimal control on my already exhausted emotions, all I could do was silently pray for a car to pass in this quiet suburban neighborhood. Eventually one did, and I would do what I did countless other mornings; I threw out my thumb, hoping to hitch a ride home. I was never fearful of hitching a ride from strangers because if they did entertain ideas of kidnapping us, I knew that after experiencing one day in my life they would promptly return us home. Upon entering the stranger's car in her nightgown, Mom would fortunately change her disposition 180 degrees like Hyde to Jekyll. Suddenly she was lovely, calm, and polite as ever as if she had been waiting for their arrival. In a low tone of voice, I began, "She has Alzheimer's, and I need a ride—"

They always interrupted me: "I understand."

They, too, were members of the secret society and knew my life without knowing me at all. After a short ride we arrived, and our day would begin as if nothing happened. Mom's short-term memory was under attack by the enemy inside her, and the slate was wiped clean five minutes after an event.

Many afternoons she threatened me by gripping my heavy dining-room chairs with both hands and screaming, "If you don't take me home, I'll throw this chair through the window!" After about an hour or two of this, she would collapse in her weapon of choice, letting me know clearly that she was angry and was not going to talk to me. I was thankful for a timeout.

Then there were the days when I was driving and would purposely stop short of the Texas signs, hoping she would not read them, but inevitably she would comment, "Why is Texas invading Pennsylvania?" or "Ya know, I never even knew parts of Philadelphia looked like this." I was happy that some of the time she believed she was in Philadelphia, lessening the guilt of my kidnapping offense. My heart would always skip a beat, knowing that awareness of her true location would trigger a fit of rage. This was a prime opportunity for the enemy to exploit, but he chose not to take it. This was not an act of benevolence but a calculating maneuver that he used often—one of retreat. He used it to relax my guard, thereby securing a surprise and devastating future assault—a common principle of warfare. Many days that assault came after I pulled into the garage and opened her car door, but, exercising her power, she refused to get out. Since it was 105 degrees outside, I begged her to come into the house so she would not dehydrate and pass out from the heat. Sometimes she would fall asleep in the car, which reset her mind, allowing me to escort her into the house. Other days she got out of the car and banged violently on the garage door, screaming, "Let me out of this prison!"

Many evenings held the same. Once I was doing the dishes after dinner when Mom, once again, decided to go home. My husband, Paul, said he would follow her. After about a half an hour, he came in without Mom.

"Where's Mom?"

"She's on the golf course, walking to Philadelphia."

He came back to get her wheelchair. With wet hands and no shoes, I flew out the door, across the street, through a neighbor's lawn, and onto the path of the private golf course, seeing Mom stomp home. I cautiously approached her.

"Hey, Mom, where ya going?"

"Home to Philadelphia!"

"Mom, Philadelphia isn't that way. It's this way."

Paul had the wheelchair, and we took her back to "prison," as she called it. Many evenings when she was angry, she would direct her wheelchair into a dark corner of the living room and pout to punish me. Her manipulating maneuver was always successful. This was my life on countless mornings, afternoons, and evenings.

These were just a few of the daily episodes that flashed through my mind during my brother's first visit when he said, "You look terrible." Considering I was battling an unseen enemy inside a person I loved twenty-four hours a day, seven days a week without real sleep while managing an angry husband, the household finances, my mother, food shopping, laundry, and providing three full-course meals a day, I thought I looked pretty darn good. I even put on makeup for his arrival. When I didn't respond to his comment, he turned his attentions toward Mom.

My brother, familiar with Mom's daily antics, would stay the weekend to give me a break, but ultimately Monday morning came, and he would leave for the airport. I would lie in bed and cry, hearing him sneak out of the house at 5:00 a.m., because when he was there I felt supported, and when he left I felt so alone, knowing I was barely holding things together. He had to sneak out before she awoke because he was her favorite child, the one she identified with and was most proud of. I was not the one she preferred. However, as God's providential order would have it, I was her lifeline, and we were somehow going to work out this relationship. The amalgam of my physical depletion and the emotional labyrinth of our relationship overwhelmed me. Every now and then I wondered how to be a good wife and daughter at the same time. I was trying my best to fulfill both roles yet failing at both.

CALLING IN REINFORCEMENTS

Initially my brother and I divided responsibilities. He had power of attorney, taking care of the finances, bills, elder-care lawyers, and real-estate agents for the ultimate sale of her house. I was to take care of Mom and her doctor appointments. Now that Mom lived with me, in between all this trauma drama, I made endless phone calls while filling out reams of paperwork to transfer power of attorney from my brother to me. Most importantly, I had to reestablish Mom's doctors, especially those who would treat her Alzheimer's disease.

Houston attracts people from all over the world to its well-known medical centers. I heard only good things about the Alzheimer's unit and was very hopeful. When we arrived at the hospital, they did not need to educate me about Alzheimer's. They knew I was well acquainted with the strategies of my formidable foe. His invasion was slow but sure footed. Unlike a human terrorist, he did not set up cells; he destroys cells. Confusing the main computer, the brain, is his lethal and crippling weapon.

Mom had cognitive testing in Philadelphia; however, the Houston doctors required a new mental baseline. Initially they did not invite me to accompany her during the testing until the therapist came out of the room, stating, "She's agitated and insulted at the simplicity of the questions and won't cooperate." I was then invited to sit in on her testing. Mom had great respect for authority figures, especially doctors, and rarely acted up in front of them.

During each visit, before the therapist entered the room to begin the test, I briefed Mom on the day, date, and year, hoping she would remember at least one of them. The testing began. "Corinne, who is this woman to my right?"

My heart screamed: *If you get any answer right, please just let it be that one!*

"My daughter."

Hearing her response was like balm to my soul. His questioning continued as to the time, date, month, year, the city she was in, how old she was, word spelling, number adding, and drawing hands on a clock to a specific time. During the test her beautiful blue eyes begged me for the answers. Although I wanted to scream the answers inside her brain, I sat in silence as she struggled, searching for the elusive responses. She failed the clock test, and could not answer any of the questions accurately. Knowing that her response was erroneous, she would add a compensating smile and comment. "I always knew the day and date when I worked."

The emotionless therapist, ignoring her comment, continued on to the next question. Mom looked at me, and I knew what she was thinking: names she screamed at me often—"traitor" or "turncoat." I knew she wanted to pass all the tests since she had always been a straight-A student. I wished I could have made her understand that it was not her fault. She was still one of the brightest in her class.

They gave a score neither of us understood, but it was not what it should be. Normally when taking a test, if you fail, you stay at the same level. Not with Alzheimer's. You were demoted. Alzheimer's never promotes anyone. He is a malicious, cold-blooded enemy whose goal is to take the person and everyone who loves her down, and he does it ever so slowly to ensure maximum suffering and heartbreak.

After the therapist finished, he led us into another room to wait for the doctor. Because I heard she was a pioneer in the field of dementia and Alzheimer's, lecturing all over the world, I anticipated a woman of great compassion. However, her debut was cold and clinical, exhibiting little kindness or friendliness. Compassion was not in her emotional vocabulary. Mom shook her hand as the doctor sat down.

"Hello, Corinne. I'm your doctor. Do you know the name of the hospital you are in right now?"

The doctor, ignoring Mom, began flipping through the medical notes, giving my mother ample time to struggle. My heart wrenched as Mom rummaged through her mind, desperately trying to find an answer for the authority figure. I immediately knew that this woman was not part of the secret society. The enemy called Alzheimer's had not touched her life or heart. She was like an analyst sitting unscathed in an office, evaluating statistics on a war that she never fought in or experienced. As Mom's silent labor became palpable, the doctor, void of emotion, slammed an invisible gavel and decreed in an adjourning tone, "She couldn't pull it up," sealing her verdict by closing Mom's folder as she had done with many others. She had seen it all before. I was hoping for a weapon to kill off or push back the enemy, but the only weapons she offered were available medications to keep Mom calm and the enemy at bay.

At first I hesitated, not wanting to give Mom any drugs until the doctor said with cold impatience, "It would give her a better quality of life." I immediately agreed. I was to increase the dosage every two weeks by 2.5 milligrams to arrive at the proper dosage. It was a slow, slow process— too slow. The first medication failed after a few months. Then there were nights when she pursed her lips in rebellion, refusing to take her meds, believing I was poisoning her. The second drug had some promise but with side effects, and we had not yet reached the right dose. I had mixed feelings about increasing the dose but was left with few options. Even though Mom was on medication, her middle-of-the-night escapades continued.

In my unrelenting attempts to brainstorm about Mom's sleep issue, I came up with the idea of taking her to a sleep center for an evaluation, hoping that part of the problem was sleep apnea. After I made all the necessary arrangements, my husband dropped us both off to spend the night. A very calm and tenderhearted technician led us to a beautiful, serene room painted with soothing colors, dotted with candles, and surrounded by Zen-type music. Mom sat in the chair as the technician instructed. Slowly, methodically, and patiently, the technician began attaching probes all over Mom's head with a gooey gel. She must have had about fifty or more probes streaming from her head, forcing her hair to stick up in many directions. She looked like the bride of Frankenstein. I kept thinking how she would have battled me if I had been attaching those probes with cold goo onto her scalp. This imaginary scene played out in my head, forcing me into the bathroom for a long, quiet, guilty laugh. When I returned, Mom continued to sit quietly like an obedient child as the technician finished her tedious task. My heart swelled with love as Mom sat there because she was always a trooper and trusted every idea I came up with to help her, no matter how crazy or foreign it was to her comprehension.

With a big smile, the woman instructed Mom in a calm, sweet, bedtime voice in concert with the serene room.

"Now, Corinne, just go to sleep, and we are going to monitor you all night in a booth outside the glass window. There are cameras, so we can see you and talk to you through the speakers."

Mom nodded her wired head in understanding.

"Donna, we have a room for you down the hall."

Although that was music to my ears, I did not want to be too far from Mom.

"If possible, I'd rather sleep next door."

"Not a problem. Here's the key."

I opened the door; silence and tranquility filled the atmosphere. It was a dream room filled again with candles, music, a shower, and my most-coveted possession: alone time. That night I thought maybe I could try to sleep. However, all during the night I kept hearing the once-calm, soft-spoken woman over Mom's loudspeaker, shouting frantically, "Corinne, stay put. Wait for me. Corinne! The probes are coming out of your head! Corinne, stop. Corinne!"

Opening doors, closing doors, quickly paced footsteps running up and down and in and out of Mom's room. I just lay there, my eyes wide open, contemplating getting up but selfishly relishing that, for this one night, I did not have to drag my war-torn body out of bed to respond. I lay there staring at the ceiling, as I did every other night, while listening to another woman fight the enemy.

After lying awake all night, I got up at 5:00 a.m. and leaned my exhausted body onto the wall of the shower. I had not enjoyed a shower in months. Most mornings I ended up quickly showering with Mom because I would get soaked leaning into the shower to wash her. Leaving her alone was never a good idea. The hot water felt nurturing to my body and soul. By six I was dressed. The woman came over my loudspeaker. In a singsong tone like a mother waking her child, the technician whispered, "Donna, it's six o clock...time to get up."

I asked myself, *Who could sleep with all the noise?*

My husband picked us up. My thought that maybe it was sleep apnea failed. What was I thinking? No, it was Alzheimer's. The enemy's military expeditions continued to sabotage my every attempt in trying to help Mom. As we drove away I mentally logged in another conquest for the enemy and another defeat for me.

My eldest cousin, whose life was organized, calm, and in control, called to suggest that I put Mom in respite care for the weekend so I could think and calmly make a decision about my next move. I knew she meant well, but there was no way my mother would stay in a respite-care center for the weekend. She was too combative. I knew I would be on the phone all weekend. Our extended family did not understand Alzheimer's. They never met him. Mom referred to him as Al and would say, "Oh, I can't remember. Al is visiting me right now." As friendly as Mom referred to him, I knew he was the enemy and was winning every battle. As I thought about my cousin's suggestion, I fantasized about going there for the weekend.

In Spite Of The Enemy

Despite the daily dramas, I was determined to make Mom's life vital and lived to the fullest. I established activities for her, incorporating them into my daily routine. Like a new mother I now donned a fully equipped diaper bag, transport chair, sun umbrella, and easy crossword books, and off in the car we would go. While driving I would blast the radio, and we would sing songs together. She would dance in her seat to the beat of Michael Jackson and enjoy my serenading solos of

Nat King Cole, Frank Sinatra, or the latest pop songs. However, she especially loved when I personalized a song by working her name, Mom, or Mommy in the appropriate places. She would get a real kick out of that, but the song she liked the best was the one I wrote for her. When I sang it she would smile as big as ever and say, "Did you write that for me?" Every time I sang it, in her mind it was the first time she heard it. These were the times when I was her hero, and they were a balm over my soul.

Our day trips varied, depending on the weather. Some days I took her clothes shopping or to the gym, where we both participated in senior water aerobics. On other days we took long wheelchair walks in the park or sat on a park bench and talked about things that we never had. She would tell me about the things she loved in nature. Clouds became a great fascination to her. Having grown up in the city, the high buildings had eclipsed their beauty. On other days I took her on her favorite outing: food shopping. I became a master at pulling the shopping cart with one hand and pushing her wheelchair with the other, making this event last three times longer. I didn't care because it kept Mom calm and busy. I included her in on the food choices and gave her items to place in the basket cradled on her lap to give her a sense of purpose. She always lit up when she saw Spanish cinnamon cookies. Like a mother wrapped around her child's finger, I would always allow them to end up in her basket, hoping to keep up her weight. We visited the ever-so-kind bread woman, who always made a fuss over Mom. Mom never remembered her from visit to visit, but she would beam from the attention and proudly retell the woman all about her father, a Sicilian bread baker, who came to this country and started a bakery making the best bread she ever ate.

I made holiday dinners, and invited friends who were good with Mom, and took photos to make it special for her. I would take her out to lunch, which she loved, except the ordering part. I would glance over at Mom scanning the menu. She could not order because the menu was overwhelming. To minimize her confusion I would engage her in our normal exchange.

"What are you getting, Mom?"

"Oh, I don't know. You decide for me."

Do you want fish or meat? Soup, salad, or a sandwich?"

"Surprise me."

I took Mom for her first facial, praying she would not act up during the treatment. The woman who I had gone to many times before was extra gentle. When we left Mom grabbed the woman's face and thanked her. I was so relieved that she enjoyed herself because normally she did not feel comfortable receiving care from a stranger. Her mother had raised her to give, not to receive.

Mom's parents were pioneers in a new country. They were hardworking Italian immigrants who started a bread bakery while raising eight children and burying the ninth. My mother, the youngest, became her mother's helper and a servant to all. Duty consumed her and unknowingly became her taskmaster. Mom defined herself through her various roles of daughter, wife, sister, and mother. Although one of the brightest among her siblings, Mom did not have the option to go to college; that opportunity was given only to her brothers, believing men had to support a family. Nevertheless, her stellar grades and work ethic ushered her front stage as the valedictorian of her high-school class. After graduation Mom began and ended her career in banking. She was organized, efficient, and completed all tasks with excellence, meeting the needs of her elderly customers beyond her job description. She raised me to be the same: efficient, organized, and a servant. Serving was in my DNA. Although taking care of Mom was challenging, it was also a privilege and came as naturally to me as breathing.

Coming from a long line of duty-filled servants, my mother never heard the words "I love you" spoken to her as a child; therefore, they were never spoken to my brother or me as children or adults. Once I asked her why she never said, "I love you." Her response was that of a servant: "If I didn't love you, I wouldn't do the things I do for you. Most people say it but never show it. I show it!" Servanthood was Mom's love language. It did not matter if the other person's love language was different. When she moved in with us, I began telling her I loved her, and after a while she began to respond with ease. In her illness I was teaching her to receive service from others while showing her a different love language: one spoken, one heard.

Our most peaceful times were in the kitchen. I would give her a small job as she gave to me as a child, such as snapping green beans. She would sit in her transport chair as we talked, prepared dinner, or dried dishes. Sometimes I was her daughter. Sometimes I was her friend. But most times I was her closest sister, Gloria, the cinnamon-bun thief, who had since died.

Once I took advantage of the situation when she thought I was her friend because, growing up, in the depths of my heart, I knew she preferred my brother to me. When three people over the years observed our family dynamics and confirmed my suspicion, it broke my heart. She gravitated toward him like steel to a magnet. I would jump through hoops, and she barely recognized, celebrated, or applauded my efforts. With all this in mind, I asked her, "Corinne, tell me about your daughter, Donna."

In a ho-hum tone she responded, "Oh, she's okay. She is very organized, efficient, a good cook, a good wife, and she gets things done. But let me tell you about my son!"

Off she went with a beaming smile into a sales pitch about her son. I just laughed, and in a moment that part of my soul began healing. Unknowingly, Alzheimer's had saved me years of therapy. I heard it straight from the source.

"Do you want to have a date with him?"

"Mom, he's my brother!"

"No, he's not. That would mean you are my daughter, and you are not my Donna."

"What's my name?"

"Donna."

"Exactly. I'm your daughter."

"No, you're not."

"Then who am I?"

"I don't know, but I think you'd be good for my son."

Round and round we would go into our daily, frustrating, cyclical monologue of Abbott and Costello's routine "Who's on First."

THOUGHTS IN MY FOXHOLE

At the end of a busy day people usually welcome the nighttime to rest and unplug from their busy lives. For me, however, nighttime was not a time of rest. The bed next to Mom's became my foxhole, where I waited for the next assault. If asked, any soldier would tell you that the dark stillness of one's foxhole becomes sacred ground. It is a time when everything in life comes into sharp focus, and you think your most honest thoughts. Since sleep eluded me, I used this time to rest my body while assessing the damage done to my marriage, my physical body, or my heart. After assessing the time spent with Mom during the day or the casualties of the day, my attentions turned to God.

Most nights I pleaded with God to take Mom home back to Him and spare me the emotional pain of placing her into a memory-care facility. However, God remained silent. Throughout my spiritual journey I have come to understand His silence. God always answers our prayers. Sometimes what we view as a lack of response is actually Him saying, "Wait" or "no." Other times it serves as reinforcement for our faith that He will accompany us through the difficult circumstances to grow our lives and characters. It can also be an opportunity to submit to His testing. In my heart I suspected it might be the latter two. I began viewing caring for Mom as being in God's love class. The classroom was my home, and the teacher, of course, remained silent during the test. The test had one question that I wrestled with daily: How will you respond to the adversity the enemy is aiming at you?

Lying there, I thought about Jesus, who, in His moment of adversity, pleaded with Father God in the Garden of Gethsemane to remove His imminent crucifixion. God did not but again remained silent. In submission, Jesus embraced pain and death, becoming the final atoning sacrifice God required to forgive the sins of mankind. Father God then resurrected Jesus, showing His acceptance of this great love sacrifice that secured victory over death for all those who believe in the sacrifice of Jesus. I meditated on this every night because to know God, one has to know His ways. I knew He is a God of the resurrection. Whenever there was a sacrifice of love, there would be a resurrection. This became the basis of my hope and confidence. Lying there, I wondered what type of resurrection He had in mind for Mom and me and when I would see it.

While reflecting on all this, I had a sobering thought: during His most difficult hour in the garden, Jesus was in God's ultimate will. I mused if my difficult situation was the center of God's ultimate will for me. My mind began walking through the scriptures. Although His imminent crucifixion would be difficult, God knew the end result would be victorious like a mother who goes through intense labor pains, resulting in the joy-filled miracle of a new life. I knew that if I kept my eyes on Jesus, I, too, would experience the priceless commodity of joy even though all I could see from my vantage point was pain and suffering (Hebrews 12:2). God is in the heart business. My faith told me that He was going to use this chapter in my life to not only change my heart but enlarge its capacity. The one thing I did not know was that in order for my heart to get bigger, it had to be broken.

One night while lying in my foxhole, the enemy launched an attack as Mom battled me from one until three in the morning. I could have literally strangled her because I was so physically spent, mentally exhausted, and emotionally stressed. In extreme frustration I began hitting myself in the head until it hurt while pleading with her to stop torturing me. After our battle ended she collapsed on the couch in the dark, where she slept with her head on my shoulder, and I loved her to pieces. I believe this polarity was part of the enlargement of my heart. One minute she broke it open and all my junk would come out and the next, unknowingly, love and compassion mended it together. Afterward I would evaluate my response to her the night before, questioning how I could have handled it better. I knew I was really yelling at the enemy, but in doing so I yelled at my mother, making the enemy's cowardly plot successful. Some of my journal entries just say, "I yelled at Mom yesterday. Oh, God, please forgive me!" God's forgiveness was always there for me to have a do over and get it right. His mercy is so great. This is how God helped me. During it all His grace carried me.

All soldiers know that privacy is at a premium within the close proximity of the foxhole. Because of the disease, Mom, unaware that I was in the next bed, began praying to God. I felt guilty listening to her private prayers yet privileged for a glimpse into the portal of her soul. She asked God's blessing for my brother and me, and she asked for guidance to do the right thing, to be a good daughter and wife. My heart broke when she demonstrated such humility. For months I would lie there listening to her talk to God or to herself of her frustrations and dreams, but mostly I listened to her take verbal stands against people who had taken advantage of her or treated her poorly over the years. I knew such a privilege came with responsibility to keep things she unknowingly revealed confidential. It was during the night hours that I learned more about the woman I only knew in her role as "Mom" that I otherwise would never have known.

As my love for Mom continued to deepen, I would lie in my foxhole, meditating on love—my limited love for her in the past and my expanding love for her now. I wondered if it was possible to love someone too much. At times the deep love I felt for her overwhelmed me to tears. It was painful and beyond my capacity to contain. If I could barely contain the depth of my love for one person, how unfathomable God's love must be to have the capacity to love billions upon billions of people since creation and not be destroyed by it. While I was thinking about God's great capacity to love, my humanity came into sharp focus. It made the passages I have read so many times in the Bible come to life as well as what Apostle Paul prayed for all people to experience: "May your roots go down deep into the soil of God's marvelous love. And may you have the power to understand as all God's people should, how wide, how long, how high, and how deep His love really is" (Ephesians 3:17–18 NLT).

I believed Mom and I were both inside God's heart, and He was going to work together all this adversity to accomplish His purposes in me, in her, and in our relationship. This season of my life would not end until He completed the necessary work. We were getting a lesson in the highest form of love, sacrificial love—the most difficult yet the most rewarding and fruitful. As I lay there contemplating the breadth and length and depth of His great love, I knew this was not just caring for Mom.

It was a high calling to love sacrificially and was worth every struggle. The reward was that, as I loved her completely, I increased my own capacity to love others.

MOTHERHOOD

When my brother arrived back in Philadelphia after we kidnapped Mom, he called to see how things were going. In the course of our conversation, he said, "Donna, Mom is now your child." My womb had never held or birthed a child, but in that moment his words fertilized the womb of my heart. The invisible mantle of motherhood was laid on me. She would become my mother-child, and through her I would experience motherhood. She became the nucleus of my life, and I was like a flying electron orbiting her with energy, propelled by love and loyalty. His statement would play out in my life and become my reality.

Motherhood never crossed my mind unless someone brought it up. I never had the desire everyone said I was supposed to have. It never appealed to me, having observed most young mothers to be too manic with their kids, thereby allowing motherhood to swallow up their identities. I also did not want to have that much control over another human being. Nor did I want to be the center of someone's universe, believing it would be all consuming, smothering, and had to hurt. After my childbearing years ended, I was happy to have escaped its grip. Nevertheless, I was like Sarah in the Bible, who was past her childbearing years but whose womb God opened up; through Mom He opened mine. For me, God could only do a deep work in my heart through motherhood—the one role that penetrates the core of a woman's being as nothing else can.

Young mothers are up most nights as their children suckle needed nutrients from their breasts. My mother-child did not draw milk from me, but the enemy drew out all the ugliness inside my character. I hated the stuff that would come out of me as the enemy tried every emotional shade in me: impatience and anger instead of longsuffering and self-control, frustration instead of kindness, pride and forcefulness instead of gentleness, all resulting in strife. Mom's mental condition challenged my heart condition the second night she began living with me in Houston.

I wheeled her transport chair into the bathroom. "Mom, it's time to take a shower."

Mom, like a defiant child, responded, "I don't want to take a shower."

For thirty minutes she battled me and finally sat cross-armed, unmovable in silent rebellion. Most mothers would pick up their rebellious thirty-five-pound children and place them in the tub, but you cannot do this with a hundred-pound adult. Exhausted emotionally and physically from the last five weeks of caring for her and her Philadelphia home and from kidnapping her two nights before, I was in no mood and shouted, "Mom, if you're not going to make a decision soon, I'm going to make it for you!" I shuddered when I heard myself. I sounded just like a Nazi mom. Was this the type of parent I would have been? She shot me a look, forcing me to examine how I had just spoken to my mother, who I am supposed to honor. Her look said, "This is why I don't want to live with you." I stood there and dropped my head in shame. Even though this disease made the simplest of tasks challenging, it was no excuse.

Anyone can be nice when things are going great. However, it is only in the presence of adversity that the real you emerges, and you come face to face with who you truly are. The adversity became a sharp instrument in God's hand, reproving, pruning, and challenging my response to the enemy. There were dual battles underway: the war I was fighting with the enemy and the war I was fighting within myself. Over time this battle drew out and exposed every raw human emotion in me, forcing me to examine each one to change it, enlarge it, replace it, or dispense of it. I had a choice, and over time I made a conscious decision to use this entire situation as a stepping stone and not a stumbling block, although there were days when I did stumble. When I did, I got back up, corrected myself, and moved forward.

To write this book I reread my journals. Since Mom's arrival into my Houston home, I hadn't spilled as much ink onto the pages of my journal as I used to, and one day's entry simply stated: "Mom hated me today." Being the bad guy in her eyes caused the most difficult days just like for any mother whose child yells, "I hate you!" I was not sure what happened the day I wrote this. I wondered if she hated me because of the shallow well of my heart and soul or if it was a day when I had to dish out tough love. I came to realize that this love was tough on both of us—tough on me because it forced me to be her parent, tough on her because she was being treated like a child by her own child.

The progression of the disease made Mom more child-like, increasing my motherly instincts. I found myself hovering over and protecting her in other people's company. I never wanted anyone around Mom without me present. I wanted to be there to preserve her dignity because many times she could not understand or hear what a person was asking or could not find a response. In those moments she would glance at me with a look that said, "Help me." I was always there to do so. One time, for example, my husband has some friends over. While there, they ignored Mom even though she was in their company for two hours. I was amazed because I just wanted them to treat her as she still mattered even though she was confused. After all, another human being was suffering. I learned that when people do not acknowledge sick people, they show the sickness of their own hearts.

Other times Mom, with the innocence of a child, said things without understanding the impossibility of her thought. One such time was at a formal dinner party given by our neighbors, Ken and LaHonda. Like a mother, I dressed Mom in her finest. Our neighbors were very sweet, patient, and understanding toward Mom, and she felt comfortable in front of them and never acted up. As we sat in their living room having a glass of wine before dinner, LaHonda mentioned something to me about our mutual neighbor across the street named Ann. Mom, trying to contribute to the conversation, thought we were talking about her neighbor in Philadelphia whose name was also Ann. I responded to Mom, trying to differentiate between the two women, "No, Mom, that's a different Ann, and, besides, she's dead."

Mom looked perplexed and said, "Again?" LaHonda and I could not stop laughing. Mom laughed too.

Mom never remembered who was dead or alive and thereby resurrected people on a daily basis. Since she was the youngest sibling, most of her family had died. It became our daily, constant, exhausting conversation and battle as she demanded to know, "Did my mom eat?" or "Where's Daddy?" At first I would patiently show her the newspaper obituaries and small Catholic funeral cards listing the name, birth, and death of the person, but Mom would knock the large pile out of my hand onto the floor, announcing, "I don't believe them." This led me to invent "the dead list." I taped it onto the refrigerator door as any mother would do when trying to reinforce lessons to their child. Now exhausted by our daily, repetitive conversation and frustrated at her inability to grasp the lesson, I would stand in front of the list, point to, and recite each name followed by an exasperated, thunderous decree, "They're dead!" Daily she would rip it down, and I would reattach it. One day she asked, "Where's Flint?"

In my frustration I yelled, "Mom, he's dead too. Mom, everybody's dead!" I got a pen and forcefully scribbled the dog's name to the bottom of the dead list.

People told me to go along with her. For me, confirming her confusion was giving in to the enemy. However, eventually I did get rid of the dead list because, through a dream one night, God told me "to respect everyone's reality." When I did, I became a master at instant storytelling in answering her questions. Two minutes later she forgot we even had the conversation. However, more importantly, I was respecting her by respecting her reality.

Respect is what all people deserve whether they know it or not.

The more childlike Mom became, the more I wanted to put her inside my womb and carry her around. Other times I wanted to crawl back inside her womb and reassume my place, where it was dark, quiet, warm, peaceful, and nourishing. A place where there was natural order. She would be my mother, and I had no responsibility to be hers.

SURRENDERING TO THE ENEMY

"There's no way you can take care of someone with Alzheimer's!" my friend Richard shouted at me across the table when he heard that I was caring for Mom in my home. He had tried to take care of his Alzheimer's-ridden mother in his home with little success, recounting every fight and corresponding battle wound with heartwrenching details. I remained silent because in my mind I wore an imaginary cape. I had worn it successfully in the past when life's circumstances demanded I push myself into twelfth gear. I knew my edge and my high level of stamina from past exploits involving my energies. However, as this war raged on, I would lie in my foxhole recalling Richard's words. The enemy's relentless attacks weakened me on three fronts: spiritually, emotionally, and physically. I felt knocked down by a turbulent wave that was tossing, tumbling, and moving me forward, making it impossible to get my footing. In response I pushed my limits full throttle, knowing that I was the last frontline before placing Mom in a home.

One time Mom had a lucid moment while I bathed her. With her head cast down, she said, "This isn't fair to you. Put me someplace." I wasn't emotionally ready for such a move. I wondered if I would ever be ready. Therefore, I ignored her comment just as she had ignored many of my concerned comments over the years.

Raised with strong Italian traditions and family loyalties, we did not put our family in nursing homes. Instead we sacrificed and cared for them, and they continued to be a part of our lives, an area of our tradition that I greatly admired. However, with each passing month, my once-robust daily prayer life was reduced to a short, simple, feeble, frustrated, and tear-filled plea: help me. Words that came from a place of desperation and fear—fear that I would literally lose my mind. I always knew my edge physically and emotionally, but I had never reached it this closely.

As I felt my body and immune system weakening, I wondered who would care for Mom if I were to get sick. Externally I was handling things, but inwardly I knew the toll this war was taking on my physical and emotional health and that if I kept at this pace, it would destroy me.

In the eighth month of Mom's stay, a friend in Houston told me about a private memory-care home without an institutional environment located thirty minutes from our home. However, I was not emotionally ready for such a move without my brother's support, but after an extremely difficult day with Mom, on October 20, 2010, I came to the edge of my edge and surrendered.

I called my brother, telling him I could not do this any-more and to begin researching similar types of homes near Philadelphia. I did not have a journal entry for that day, but on October 30, 2010, after the fact, my entry was one of regret, ending with, "Motherhood, how crazy are these emotions, they are devouring me and my love is bleeding. Today I surrendered." I wished I could take it back and try one more time, but I knew the result would be the same. The battle reports that lay before me were undeniable. The enemy had taken too much ground, and I had failed in my mission to protect and defend Mom from the fate that awaited her. Although unsuc-cessful, I was satisfied that I had tried my best, pulled out every stop, and pushed myself beyond my limits. My arsenal was empty; my marriage was on life support, my health a wreck, my emotions distressed, and my woman-power depleted.

We put our house up for sale a third time. It was God's timing because after two prior attempts, the house sold in one month; it was November 15, 2010. I was so excited to leave Houston and all it represented. It was never home, nor would it ever be. Unaware of the move, Mom sat impatiently while I packed my breakables and personal items before the movers' arrival. Our departure date was December 31, 2010. The plan was for Mom and me to fly out to Mom's home in Philadelphia, and my husband would stay, manage the movers, and drive the cars back from Houston.

My husband drove us to the airport and carried our luggage onto the sidewalk as I helped Mom into her transport chair. As I reached up to his six-foot frame to kiss him good-bye, he stood erect and rigid, his heart impenetrable, his anger tangible. He was angry that he had to manage the movers himself. He also had to drive two cars from Houston to Philadelphia. I suggested he have a friend of ours sell one car in Houston and drive one back, but he said no. As he walked away from us toward the car, I felt relieved knowing that I was temporarily released from my failing role as wife and able to focus on my failing role as daughter. As I watched him pull away, my mind recounted the countless times I unpacked and packed alone in other countries, turning our house into a home while he was at work. I considered caring for Mom my work, except I never received a salary, a vacation, a bonus, time off, or an atta girl. Unable to sort through the injustice of it all, I let it go and pushed Mom's chair forward into the airport.

I led a now-medicated Mom, like a small child, onto the plane. She did not know where we were going or from where she was leaving or why. I held her hand as we took off, and she fell fast asleep. Looking at her, I wished I could sleep, too, but instead I began interrogating myself about the upcoming stages of this battle. *Where will I get the emotional strength to place Mom into a memory-care center? Where will I get the physical strength to manage an interstate move, empty and sell Mom's old house, visit and select a memory-care facility, set up Mom's new home, buy and set up our new house, begin doctoring my health, and function in my new role as Mom's advocate on minimal sleep? Moreover, how can I do all this and be a good wife and daughter at the same time?* My mind swirled by the unknown, I wiped my tears, blocked the future out of my thoughts, and rested my head on the window and my mind in the hum of the airplane. I wished I could sleep, but sleep continued to evade me. Staring at the white slate of clouds, I reflected on the past ten months.

I had difficult seasons in my life before, but this was, without question, the most difficult, survived only by God's grace. Although my marriage suffered casualties, and my husband was continually angry with me, I was thankful to him for making it possible for me to care for Mom at home for as long as I did. I was thankful to my cousin Marlene, who always called, guiding me from her experience with her mother's dementia. I was thankful to my brother and my friend Kenny, who faithfully called daily, listening to me vent, cry, or lie, insisting that everything was going well. I would take the phone into the bathroom while tending to Mom not to miss one call because they were my emotional lifeline. They made me feel less alone, and without them I knew I would have imploded into a complete emotional breakdown.

I then thought about the daughter in Italy, who, two years earlier, had led her mother through the Italian food market. I did not feel strong like her but felt more like a defeated and wearied soldier flying home from a battle that I had lost. I was fragile physically and emotionally, and like a soldier, I had become a different person. I did not have any visible wounds, but my wounds, like those of many soldiers, were in my heart. I wondered why they gave soldiers a purple heart for physical wounds but nothing for their emotional wounds. What color was more deeply saturated and passionate than purple? There was none. Therefore, there were no emblematic honors for the emotionally wounded. Intrinsically I understood that if my heart had become small, hardened, and angry, God's work was still undone. My heart, however, had become enriched and fearless in the face of the enemy. By this I knew that God had pinned onto my heart not a medal but His love. This emblem of honor is not something I could keep in a box but something I would inadvertently display as I lived my life. I was now a different person. No matter how beaten down the soldiers of everyday life may appear, if their hearts were enlarged by whatever battle they found themselves in then God used their battles for His ultimate will—to make them more into His image, one of love and compassion.

JANUARY 1, 2010– MAY 24, 2010

HOME AT LAST

My brother picked us up at the airport and drove us to Mom's row house in Philadelphia. I wondered what her response would be when she arrived at the place she had been walking to for the past ten months. We opened the door; she walked in, sat down, dropped her head on the couch, and took a nap. After ten months of intense arguments, hand-to-hand combat, and chasing her down suburban streets, I expected her to be excited to be home. I expected some jubilation or a hug of appreciation. No, the enemy inside her put her right to sleep. He is malevolent, ignoring every attempt to please, reward, or make anything enjoyable, using every opportunity to disappoint and destroy any ounce of joy or celebration.

The next day my brother, Mario, and I began visiting memory-care communities in and near Philadelphia. With every one I walked into, I felt sick to my stomach, not able to imagine Mom there—alone. Mom did not do well alone.

Raised with seven siblings, she always had a companion. She always asked me, "Who will be coming with me?"

Mom always wanted family companionship. Hiring a companion for her had not worked in the past and would not work now. She would not remember the individual from hour to hour or day to day, but family she remembered. This disease could not touch that memory so deeply rooted in her soul.

Since we could not find satisfaction with the care centers we visited, I contacted aplaceformom.com, and they set up additional places for us to visit. Every time we eliminated a place, we kept getting further and further from where we were planning to live. We then went to visit a home near my brother's house, two hours away from Philadelphia, in central New Jersey. It was a private home, caring for about fourteen people with memory issues. Because it was a house, it did not have an institutional atmosphere, and Mom would have her own room. At the time finding a place that participated in Medicare was not a priority. The priority was finding a place where Mom could feel comfortable and where I could have a small measure of peace to try to regain my health, my life, and my marriage.

Until her move-in date, I lived with Mom on the first floor of her Philadelphia home. During that time she slept on the couch as I lay awake on a cot right next to her so she would not fall off the couch. On the morning of January 25, she woke to a deluge of rain. I thought this was an appropriate metaphor as my heart, mind, and emotions were flooded with sadness. Mom looked so beautiful that day, but inside I knew the enemy was slowly erasing her personality. How much longer would she know me?

Many call this disease "the long good-bye." I began thinking of it as a soul eraser.

MEMORY-CARE HOME NUMBER ONE

Mario picked us up, and we drove to have lunch at her new home. Mom ate, unaware of where she was or what was happening. After lunch they tried to include her in the activities, but Mom, refusing to be treated like a child, pushed the lined drawing and the crayons away. My husband, my brother, my niece, and I set up her room by hanging photos and unpacking her clothes. There was a bed, a chair, and an armoire for her clothes. The room was very small to discourage her from staying inside it and to encourage her to socialize in the main activities living/dining room. My niece made a beautiful memory scrapbook of family photos. It remained in Mom's room, becoming a satisfying activity as we pointed to a photo and she would correctly identify members of her family.

That day my challenging job was to contain my tears and prevent myself from unraveling. Emotionally, this transition was more difficult for me than caring for her in my home. In my mind, this day meant I failed at caring for Mom. I could not care for her and retain my health, my sanity, and my marriage at the same time. The thought of leaving her to the care of others wrenched my insides as nothing ever had and like nothing ever has.

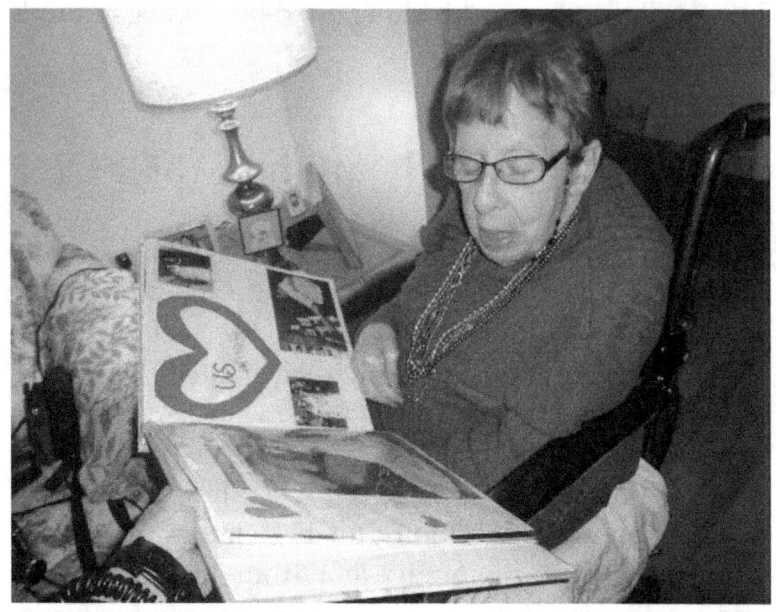

Mom exercising her memory by looking at the family album made by her granddaughter.

The home had a two-week rule, meaning that we could not contact Mom for two weeks so she could become acclimated to her new surroundings. I was to call the manager at seven every night for a full report. During these two weeks I went through the motions of looking for a new house with my husband, but, inside, my concerns for Mom monopolized my thoughts. I lived for 7:00 p.m., but their version of a "full report" was less than what I needed to hear. The manager told me Mom's first day was believing that she was in her own home and that her sister Gloria was going to be very angry at all these people in the house. Eventually she made friends with a woman named Connie. They dubbed them "Bonnie and Clyde" since the two of them would stand by the front door conspiring ways to escape.

Finally, the long two weeks were over, and we all went to see Mom. I walked into the living room; my eyes weaved through the other residents in the room to find her. I asked my brother, "Where is she?" When he pointed her out, my heart hit rock bottom, and I crashed into tears. I did not recognize her. She did not look the way I left her. Her hair was disheveled and oily. Mom had oily hair that needed washing every two days. House rules called for hair washings twice a week. I knew they could not spend the individual time with her as I did, but it still upset me. After caring for Mom twenty-four/seven, I knew her inside and out and could tell that she was uncomfortable in her heart, wishing for family companionship. I had been her companion for the last year. She was sitting on the edge of her chair, ill at ease, observing everyone as if she were at a party and knew no one. I felt like a failure, wishing I could have saved her from this fate. I just hugged her and sobbed. My heart continued to ache and break, and I was feeling emotionally and physically sick inside with no relief in sight. I did not want her to feel alone, unloved, abandoned, or betrayed as others had made her feel in her lifetime. As we drove two hours back to Philadelphia, I planned my next visit to see Mom.

My husband and I now lived temporarily in Mom's city row house while looking for a house of our own. During the week my husband kept moving us forward in looking at houses. Outwardly I went through the motions, but inwardly I did not care because my priorities had shifted, and my thoughts and concerns were for Mom. My husband wanted to live in the city of Philadelphia. Now I wanted to live in New Jersey near Mom. No homes suiting our needs became available in either state. My husband told me we had to make a decision soon since we had a time limit on our storage. Every area of my life was in flux, and my head, heart, and emotions were a moving landscape. My desire was for some area in my life to stop changing and moving so I could gain some traction and feel in control. For me, the easiest and most practical solution was to live in Mom's old row house, pay the storage fees, and save money until things with Mom played out. My husband did not like my idea, so we purchased too big a house a few blocks from my mother's old house. A neighborhood that was once my home and the landscape of my youth had become a graveyard of pain-filled memories. I was literally sick to my stomach about this decision but had little voice or footing weighed against all the inconvenience and upheaval this had caused in his life.

BUYING, SELLING, AND RENOVATING HOUSES

Mom's house was now up for sale. As a young girl I had always wondered who would clean out this huge house, spanning multiple generations where my parents and grandparents saved everything for "when you would *not* need it one day." The moment I had thought about throughout my whole life was here. My brother's schedule was busy with his job and family, so emptying the house of Mom's personal possessions was my daunting responsibility. Every time I walked into the house, memories flooded my heart. Never knowing where to start, I wandered from room to room, ending up on the steps in tears. My husband was always prompting me to empty it for a quicker sale. I knew he was right, but again his advice did not take into account my emotional state. My paralysis would last over a year.

A few blocks away, we lived among unpacked boxes. Our 1850s row house became an albatross demanding my energy to transform it from a house to a home. I never did succeed because my heart was not in it. It was not a place of refuge. It was just a place where I refreshed my suitcase. I was either preparing to pack to go see Mom or unpacking to sand, spackle, or paint. My physical health was slow in returning, and I had just found out I had Lyme disease and candida on top of adrenal exhaustion and hypothyroidism. My sleep patterns were only up to two solid hours a night as the doctor continued to reestablish balance in my adrenal system. Woven in between all this was menopause.

My husband's constant complaint was that I was not "present." His comment fluttered in my mind like an ATM machine processing a transaction. All I heard was that he needed to make a withdrawal, oblivious to the fact that I was bankrupt. No, I was not present. I felt beaten down and defeated. No matter how hard I tried, I still failed at my two most important roles as a wife and daughter. Emotionally I was in crisis: surviving something I had never known before, mystified that he could not comprehend or empathize with me. He was disconnected from my reality. In this extended season in my life, I saw others as either helping me or hindering me. I was unable to meet anyone else's needs; I was too busy failing at meeting my own. To escape my life I would fantasize about what it would feel like to be me without any defining roles and corresponding responsibilities.

The emotional and physical stress slowly began to take its toll. Many mornings I would wake up, take a shower, and get dressed with an endless list in my mind of things that needed attention. I had my pick: to help my husband paint, hang wallpaper, clean, set up newly unpacked boxes into the finished rooms, or shop for window treatments or to go to the doctor. Instead I found myself curled back into bed in tears, sick to my stomach, wishing I could unplug from my life. I was depressed, missing Mom so desperately that my insides physically ached, diminishing my appetite for everything. Every attempt I made to gain some control or balance over my mind and emotions failed. After a crying session, my husband said, "You're not what your Mom needs right now."

Intellectually, I knew he was right, but my heart silently screamed back, *But she is what I need right now!*

My friend Maria told me to get into a support group. However, the last thing I wanted to do was use my limited energies to exchange battle stories and have someone needier than I suck me dry. I could not take care of one more person.

I just wanted someone to remove my heartache, and I knew no one could but God. I thought His deep work in my heart had ended when I left Houston. However, God's excavation continued because I felt the pain of Him digging and uprooting the depths of my heart and soul even further. Since His work was ongoing, I knew my pain would stop not when I wanted it to but when God was finished performing His open-heart surgery on me.

At the core of my faith, I held on to the hope that whenever there was a sacrifice of love and a death to the less desirable qualities of the self, there would be a resurrection in my spirit that would manifest in my life.

The only time my mind, heart, and emotions were at peace away from Mom was during my brother's weekly visits with her because I knew she was with family. He told me that after lunch they sat on the couch together, and she would fall asleep on his lap. He would just sit there and cry. Even though these visits were difficult for him, I was relieved that she was not alone and did not feel abandoned or forgotten.

When my brother was not there, I would call her. "Hi, Mom, what are you doing?"

On the days when the enemy retreated, her response broke me wide open: "We are having a catch with a balloon; this is what they do with old people." Although she did not know her age any longer, Mom never considered herself old. She always read, had a curiously sharp mind, loved to dance, and had a young spirit. Other times when I called, she was incoherent, further mounting my desperation because distance prevented me from comforting her. I was powerless.

The first time I returned home to Philadelphia from visiting Mom, I began sharing about my last three days with my husband, but he interrupted me to say he did not want to hear about my time with Mom. He was tired of hearing it. My response was to shut down, punch my imaginary time clock, and begin spackling, sanding, and painting while resentfully remembering all his second family dramas I listened to over the years and all the trenches

I jumped into for him and with him. I had fought the enemy the last three days and had no energy to fight my husband, knowing a ceasefire was highly unlikely.

Every few days I checked on Mom's row house a few blocks away from my new residence. This neighborhood was my home; Mom's presence had always been my refuge, anchor, and basecamp while living overseas. Now it was just a shell of what it used to be. I felt like I was walking in a graveyard among dead memories of my past life. Everywhere I turned I saw ghosts of family members amid a culture of strangers who now claimed it as home. The feeling was both familiar and foreign.

While I was walking, the neighborhood church bells rang—a comforting sound of home. I bumped into a neighbor of over fifty years and mentioned how the church bells were such a fond memory from my childhood. She agreed and told me that the new influx of yuppiedom complained to the pastor to curtail the church bells because the sound woke their children in the morning. We concurred that the once-rich character of the neighborhood was now an empty remnant of its former days. After we parted, I recalled when my brother would call me in Houston and hold up his cell phone to share the church-bell melody then we would talk about how much we loved their sound. Now when they rang, instead of the deep, rich, satisfying tones bathing my heart and soul with comfort, sadness engulfed me. Sadness became my constant companion. Out of all the emotions in life, sadness, for me, is one of the most difficult. It is like a heavy blanket thrown over your insides, making it impossible to get out from under its weight. There is nothing you can do about it; it just is.

VISITS BEGIN

Visiting Mom became the highlight of my week not only to see her but also to still my emotional turmoil. I would pack my bags, vitamins, journal, Mom's nail polish kit, scissors, hair dye, and other necessities for a three-day visit and a sleepover at my brother's house. The drive was two hours long, and I could not get there fast enough. Every time I entered the memory-care home, my eyes raced for Mom. One time I walked in, and she was in a circle, playing ball. Immediately our eyes met. She got a huge smile on her face and began getting up to come to me, but I got there first. "I was just sitting here feeling so lonely for my family, and you walked in that very second."

Knowing she was feeling this way when I was not there caused my soul to ache. Most times when I got there, she was finishing breakfast, playing bingo, napping, having physical therapy, or exercising in her chair along with her new friends. I would get right in the middle and help the activities director until there was a break for us to have alone time.

Unfortunately, Mom's room was on the second floor, so we had to take the elevator. This particular morning I was still trying to find a level of comfort with this arrangement, and my emotions were particularly raw and volatile. While I was dying her hair, she asked, "What's on your mind?" She knew me just as well as I knew her. Even in her failing mental state, her intuition was still sharp. The disease could not touch this area deep in her spirit. However, I knew that she could not help me, so I just responded, "Nothing."

After showering her, in the white noise of the blow dryer, I thought about how difficult it was to take care of a sick person who was not aware of her illness because it forces you to be your own comfort and your own counsel. Having to be my own counsel and encourager was most difficult because my reservoir was desperately low. Inside I wanted to unload my painful emotions onto her and have her make it all better as she always had in the past when she was well. While putting on her shoes, I recalled a time when we were making the bed together in Houston. I lost control over my emotions and burst out crying. Believing I was a friend, Mom asked what was wrong. Desperate for her wisdom, I explained my dilemma of my ill mother living with me, but she did not know she was ill and how stressful it was for me and how upset I was all the time. Mom, unaware she was speaking of herself, said, "I'm sorry. That's a hard one, especially if they are stubborn." From this experience I knew that I could not get solace from her anymore. Words from Mom that used to ease my pain would never come again.

"Mom, your hair looks nice. Let's get out of here." I bundled her up and decided to take her onto the walking path that surrounded a large lake near the memory-care center for some fresh air.

While I was driving, a voice in my head spoke clearly, "Just keep going straight. Kidnap Mom again. You know how to do it. Take her away." The thought made me feel empowered and in control—a feeling that I had not felt for years. "Care for her so you are no longer emotionally upset and the hell with everyone else!" At record speed, my mind raced, calculating every detail from diapers to a place to live, but I caught myself, realizing that the enemy had infiltrated my thoughts. I was entertaining crazy thoughts that I never thought I would think. In that moment I understood why people go to the grocery store and never go home again. I totally got it. It reminded me of something my mother always said: "Don't judge me until you have walked in my shoes." Desperate emotions bring people to desperate thoughts, resulting in desperate actions.

I pushed Mom's wheelchair, forcing it upward amid grass covered in three-day-old snow and ice onto the clean pavement around the lake. Having felt in control, even briefly, magnified my powerless position, and once again tears streamed down my face. Mom interrupted my emotional wrestling match by complaining about the cold, so I curtailed our walk, realizing I needed that walk more than she did. The cold winter wind felt healing as it blew through my tired mind. We got in the car and returned to her home. After dinner I did crossword puzzles with her tablemates and prepared her for bed. After she fell asleep I left reluctantly and drove to my brother's house thirty minutes away and repeated this for three days then returned to Philadelphia two hours away to rehabbing an 1850s row house.

TWO DIRECT HITS

Getting comfortable with her new home had its challenges. My weekly visits continued for another four months. They were vital in my role as advocate but like any new mother I second guessed every decision I made on her behalf. During that time I tried my best to trust the staff and embrace this new arrangement, but the enemy marshaled his forces against me. Two such occasions stand out in my mind because Alzheimer's used two of his favorite contrasting weapons. Any military theorist would agree that contrasting weaponry laced with the element of surprise is most effective.

His first weapon was one of retreat, securing 100-percent accuracy. This method of staying just under the radar allowed Mom to realize part of the truth—that her children placed her in a home against her wishes—but not the full truth—that the enemy made caring for her at home impossible and that he was, in fact, culpable. This was one of those times.

After spending a pleasant morning at the home together, I told Mom we were going shopping to buy her some new pants. In anticipation of a great day, I strapped on her seatbelt, loaded the wheelchair in the trunk, and got into the car. As I reached for my seatbelt, Mom, looking down at her hands, spoke softly and clearly, every word laced with humility. "I never imagined I'd end up in a place like this." The one thing that I never wanted to hear was the thing she just said. Her words detonated an emotional grenade inside the car, and her simple comment unraveled me. It was an unexpected and difficult moment, one that I could not escape. I could not move forward or backward. Everything in me stood still. I sat motionless. My heart pounded as if an interrogation light burned overhead.

Most days she thought she was at work or at home, questioning why the neighbors were in her house. As crazy as that was, it was better than her knowing what I had done—put her into a home against her wishes—but this day, this moment, she knew the truth. The enemy achieved a direct hit by retreating long enough to uncover my cover. When I looked over at her, she looked like my small child, only four-foot-eight, her head cast down, her tone and posture ones of submission. She sat power-less, resigned to my authority over her even though in my mind she was still my authority. My mind desperately searched for an answer but to no avail, so I responded to her comment with a question.

"Where do you want to be?"

"Home."

"You can't climb the steps, you wander, you don't sleep all night, you forget to eat, and you are incontinent."

"I'm a pest."

"No, Mom, it's the disease, not you. We love you."

I cried while hugging and kissing her repeatedly. She did not respond or look at me, but I knew what she was thinking: *If you loved me, I wouldn't be here.*

Mom never had a high opinion of herself, no matter how I tried to boost her self-esteem over the years. I detested the fact that this situation, this moment, cemented her erroneous belief. I felt beyond horrible controlling another person's life to his or her discontent. This moment con-firmed what I had always thought about the role that I never wanted; motherhood had to hurt and did hurt. In retrospect I wished I could have pressed a pause button to compose my emotions and think of the perfect response. To this day I still do not know what that would be. We sat in silence for what seemed like an eternity. My decision to place her in this home ruled over her wishes to be home with us. The enemy took away her voice and, along with it, her heart's desire. I hated this moment, and it still haunts me to this day.

The second weapon in the enemy's contrasting arsenal was showing himself as an overt and pernicious assailant, assaulting her dignity with full guns blazing. It began as a normal day, March 15, 2010. I was driving from my brother's house, excited to spend the day with Mom. As usual, I raced in.

"Where's Mom?"

"She wanted to sleep late. She's still in bed."

"Can I have the key to her room?"

They locked everyone's bedroom doors on the outside, preventing one resident who roamed into everyone's room to steal things. The doors, however, were able to open from the inside. Rosemary rummaged through a host of keys, searching for Mom's. "Ya know, I'll just come up with you and let you into your Mom's room because I have to get something out of the laundry." The second floor was a large rectangle lined with a hallway accessing about ten bedrooms. In the center was a living room with a large flat-screen television, a bathroom, a small office, and a laundry room. I chose Mom's room to be across from the large bathroom, making it most visible and a short walk during the night to reduce her risk of falling. Slowly I was becoming comfortable with this private home. Getting to know the aides made my heart a bit calmer. Rosemary and I chatted and laughed in the elevator on the way up and, as always, I was excited to see Mom to do her morning care. The elevator doors opened to a pile of feces. With no emotional response, I said, "Oh."

Rosemary replied, "I'll get it."

We stepped over the pile, and again without any emotional response I looked to my left, and there stood a woman covered everywhere in feces in a panic, unable to speak, spinning in circles in confusion with *Reader's Digest* papers stuck to her hands. While Rosemary was en route, in a surreal, Hitchcockian nanosecond, I realized the woman was my mother. A maelstrom of emotions threw me into action, and I grabbed Mom before Rosemary did. "I have her," I said and pulled her into the shower.

Rosemary began opening all the windows on the second floor to relieve the odor. Trying to hold her steady with one hand while struggling to remove her soiled nightgown with the other before sitting her down in the shower, I kept repeating, "It's okay, Mom; it's okay, it's okay..." and began scrubbing her from top to bottom. Rosemary stuck her head into the bathroom,

"Do you need help?"

"No."

"Okay, Donna, I'll pick up the pile in front of the elevator, but I have to get back downstairs; we are short a person today. I'll send someone up later to clean up."

I did not want anyone to tend to Mom in this state. Apparently, she had gotten up, did not put on her eyeglasses, and roamed the large, square hallways in search of the bathroom located across from her room. Not finding the bathroom, she became frantic because she was unable to control the effects of her laxative. She held on to the chair rail and walls for support, ending up back in the only opened room. There lay the *Reader's Digest*, and she ripped out pages, attempting to clean herself. While I was scrubbing under her fingers and toenails, my mind shrieked in anger, *This would not have happened if she were with me!* I kept repeating to Mom through tears, "It's okay, Mom; it's okay," desperately wondering how it would be. Mom, distressed and confused, sat lifeless, staring vacantly into space. I dried, powdered, and dressed her. I kissed and hugged her, crying the whole time, but

Mom remained despondent. I had never seen her that way, and nothing I did penetrated the havoc the enemy had unleashed on her.

I took her down to breakfast, but she did not eat. I sat her on the couch with the other women, where she fell fast asleep, exhausted from the trauma. Later that day she would remember nothing—the one good thing about this horrible disease for her—but unfortunately for me, I did not have a delete button. Rosemary and I decided Mom needed to be on the first floor for closer monitoring.

I then went back upstairs; the elevator doors opened to the cold winter air carried in by the open windows. No one was there. The elevator doors closed behind me. I stood there for a moment shell shocked, viewing the damage from the enemy's blatant and audacious attack. The silent cold air was deafening and haunting. Emotional tremors reverberated in my heart, thwarting my tears. I began searching for cleaning supplies then, on my hands and knees in silent devastation, began scrubbing the walls and the crevices of the wooden floors. I did not want anyone else to do it. Her dignity had become undone, and I was preventing further unraveling. Any emotional ground I gained over the past few months with this home and its staff had been devoured by the enemy within minutes.

That evening during the ride to my brother's house, my emotions still numb, I blasted the radio, attempting to drown out the images of the day like an endless reel playing in my mind.

MAY 25, 2010–
DECEMBER 31, 2010

MOVING DAY

A s I mentioned before, the home where Mom presently lived did not participate in Medicaid. We were hoping that they would become a participant in the time that Mom lived there, but it never materialized. Therefore, we had to move her again. Apprehensive about another change, my brother and I searched for another home and found one ten minutes closer to his house that did participate in Medicaid. It was an assisted-living facility with a special one-floor area for memory-care housing with about twelve to eighteen residents. Mom would have her own room consisting of a bathroom, a large bedroom/living room, and a small kitchenette. We purchased a new couch, and I took something from every floor of her three-story row home and set up her room a few days prior with furniture, artwork, and family photos. It was a downsized replica of her oldest and dearest son, 1011. The best part was that she and I would have privacy; I could sleep there if I needed to, and there was a small refrigerator for my food.

May 25, 2010, was the day I was to pick up and relocate Mom to her new home. I arrived, finding her napping outside on the deck with the other women. Because my health and sleep were slow in returning, I functioned from a place of deficit. I felt ill equipped to manage the day. My emotions were brittle and on the fringe of my control. Instead of waking her up to go, I vacillated in the dining room, watching her sleep. My mind was readying itself, knowing I had to begin again to find a new level of comfort with a new cast of characters and new house rules. One of Mom's favorite aides approached, telling me how much he would miss Mom and began telling me stories of their interactions. I lost all restraint and began sobbing uncontrollably. Wrapping his arms around me, he assured me everything was going to be fine. Embarrassed by my lack of self-control, I just nodded my head in agreement, wanting to believe his words while wishing my brother were there to go through this day with me. I felt weak and inept, so I did what I learned to do when feeling this way; I moved forward, woke her up, and headed to her new home for lunch.

MEMORY-CARE HOME NUMBER TWO

We arrived as if it were our first day at school. After lunch we sat in the activities room, where I tried introducing Mom to the other men and women. Mom was polite but did not want anything to do with any of "the old people in the room," constantly saying, "Let's go" or "Let's hit the road." I wanted to go, too, and take her home. I wished I were rich so I could have two nurses caring for Mom in her own quarters attached to my home. Instead we went into her room, hoping to find some level of comfort.

Thankfully, this home did not have any two-week rule when I was unable to see her like the first home did. Therefore, for the next three nights, I lay awake on her couch, waiting to instruct her to the toilet's location. I placed sensor nightlights everywhere, fearing a reoccurrence of what happened before. For those three days I mostly tended to Mom's needs. During the day I observed her daily routine and studied the aides and the residents who would become Mom's second family. I was looking to find reassurance and ground my emotions. Since exhaustion eroded my patience level, I was happy to study the aides, who modeled for me how to be more patient with Mom. Although most residents could not communicate clearly, they could still understand. The aides waited patiently until the residents found a way to make their desires known. They did not treat them as if they were stupid, just mentally handicapped. In simple daily exchanges, the residents felt loved and respected.

On the third day the memory-care unit manager said to me, "Ya know, Donna, you're allowed to have a life." Her words hit me as if I were hearing another language. Since childhood Mom laced guilt into many of my decisions that were separate from her desires and traditional blueprint for me. Although I lived a full life, I always knew I was not the daughter she had always longed for. Her words of disapproval continually overshadowed my life choices. She was the voice inside my head. Events that other parents would find normal and celebrate, like backpacking through Europe at twenty-one or taking nude figure drawing classes, displeased her. The decisions of mine, however, that bothered her most were leaving her home at twenty-two, as an unmarried woman, for an apartment of my own, dating men who were not Italian, and buying my first house at the age of thirty-one as a single woman; the list, in her mind, was extensive. If she did not approve, she labeled me rebellious, but I did it anyway, struggling to remain true to my own personal growth and freedom. Although she raised me to be independent, whenever I exercised my independence, I paid a high price. This was the reason she never "liked" me. I wrote my own script and did not follow her traditional plan. Although I lived my life in spite of her disapproval, I continually wrestled with one question: Where did she end, and where did I begin? I truly needed to hear the words the manager spoke to have a life, but implementing them was foreign to me. The permission or blessing I had longed for my whole life came about thirty years too late, given by the wrong person at the most inopportune time. I wondered how to live my life when my inner world was in constant turmoil at seeing Mom suffer this way.

On the morning of the fourth day, I released my care of Mom to others, took the manager's advice, and drove back to Philadelphia.

Surrendering Territory

The following week I returned for my first visit to the new memory-care facility. Walking into her room, I met one of Mom's caretakers. She was a very gregarious woman, full of energy. I always asked the aides I met along Mom's journey if this was a job to them or a calling. Before they answered, I knew the answer, having observed not only their skills but also their hearts' intentions. For this aide it was a calling, and she knew it. With a big smile, she began telling me, "Donna, your mom is so funny. I was trying to shower her last night, and all she wanted to do was dance! So we danced and danced." Outwardly, I smiled back, but my heart screamed with jealously: "That was *my* dance, *my* moment, *my* memory, *my* privilege!"

When Mom lived with me and she was not battling me, showering time became a fun outlet. Many times Mom wanted to dance; we would dance and joke around, and she would say, "I don't know who's crazier, me or you!" Releasing her to the care of others was extremely difficult to impossible for me, making me feel expendable. Here was a woman who took care of everyone, and now strangers cared for her. Many considered caring for her a job, but for me it was a privilege.

As Alzheimer's continued robbing me of experiences with Mom, I wondered if this is what mothers go through as they drop their children off at preschool. Other people experience precious moments that mothers miss. Mom was learning how to relinquish her independence and control, allowing others to care for her, while I was learning how to let go of Mom's care to others. I was not very good at it, nor would I ever be.

In my continued role as advocate, I set up a meeting with Mom's new neurologist. Since her previous neurologist had decreased her evening antianxiety medication to the lowest dosage of 2.5 milligrams, I asked if we could try eliminating it altogether. Although the medication kept her calm, it also had adverse side effects, rendering it both a blessing and a curse. He agreed, but after one day the enemy reemerged, and I received a call that Mom was combative, biting and pulling the hair of three aides attempting her morning care. They had no choice but to restart her medication. I left home immediately. Upon my arrival, I found Mom still in bed. Kneeling next to her bed and seeing the black and blue handprints on her arms, flooded my mind with images of the aides trying to restrain the enemy within. Wrapping my arm around her, I kissed her awake. Her eyes opened. "Hi, Mom! Come on; get up so we can go out today."

Mom just lay there; her beautiful blue eyes studied my face, and she said, "I'm disgusted with my life. It's not worth living anymore." Lucid moments like this wrenched my heart like nothing else. I never knew how to respond except with the faith that I was holding on to.

"Mom, if God has you here on this earth then you still have purpose," but Mom remained silent. My only attempt at comforting her was getting under the covers, and like two spoons we would nap for a while then talk and joke around until her memory and mood reset.

For the next few months, I arrived weekly at the home, bogged down with the weight of my handbag, bundles of deposable panties, my food, and supplies for Mom, and began my walk down the ninety-foot-long hallway. How I hated that hallway ending with a locked door to the memory-care area. Each step reverberated exhaustion throughout my body while I was wondering, *What happened while I was not here? Will Mom still know I am her daughter? Will she be in a good mood? Will she be combative for the entire day? Was she combative toward the staff as they tried to care for her? Will I be able to take her out today? Will I see the progress of the disease? On the other hand, will the enemy's takeover continue to be slow, clandestine, and painful?*

As I walked into her room, my eyes quickly scanned it, and when I found her, I always had the same screaming thought, *She doesn't belong here. She belongs home with family.* However, because Alzheimer's is an unrelenting enemy, she was there, held as his prisoner.

Although having her live apart from me broke my heart, I was thankful that she could still communicate with me. I never knew when this disease would erase her speech and communication. Once when feeling desperate, I hugged her so tightly that she said in a meager attempt to comfort me, "I'm okay. I'm okay."

I responded, "Maybe I'm not."

Even in her illness, she sensed my desperation. In that moment I told her what a privilege it was to be her daughter and how I appreciated all that she had taught me, detailing each thing. Mom exclaimed, "Did I teach you all that?" Having lived her life so bound to duty, she never stepped back to applaud and celebrate all she had accomplished in her role as mother. No matter what the enemy stole from Mom, he could never touch all the seeds she had sown, all the fruit she bore, and all that she meant to us.

Thanksgiving was the first holiday when I had to go and pick her up to spend the day together. It felt so unnatural, but the most difficult part of a holiday was taking her back to the home. When I got her coat, she said, "Back to the hospital." The enemy's retreat gave Mom momentary clarity. When we arrived, I readied her for bed, again the enemy retreated, and Mom began voicing her complaint. "I don't like strangers taking care of me. I don't like not being independent."

"Mom, these people take care of you while Mario and I are not available." She did not respond. Again our decision of placing her in a home ruled over her heart's desire to be in her own home. My heart broke, wishing I could give her what she wanted in this last season of her life. The enemy relished in his control over me by forcing me to relinquish my care of Mom to others.

The next day I took Mom back to the family beach house. She said, "I don't feel right."

Kneeling in front of her chair, I asked, "Explain to me what you are feeling."

"I don't know. I just feel confused."

My heart broke even more, if that were possible. I never knew how to respond, although the truth was ever-present in my mind. *Mom, you have a disease that confuses you and is deteriorating your brain and your memory and all your basic functions.* Since the truth was heartwrenching to say and devastating to hear, I defaulted to the language of silence just as the woman in the card store did years earlier.

Then she killed me off and said, "I feel lonely a lot of the time. I look around, and I don't see anyone I know—I don't see family. I am alone, and I feel lonely."

My love for her became the bridge connecting me to her pain, her suffering, her aloneness, and her loneliness. Seeing her suffer was emotionally painful for me. I wished I could take her disease onto myself believing it would hurt me less. I knew the impossibility of this but it was my mind's solution to escape my pain. The reality was that I had surrendered precious territory and could no longer rescue her. I quelled my emotions and responded the way I usually did in moments when words eluded me—with hugs and kisses. She understood this language best. It made us believe everything would be fine. After this episode I wrote a two-page healing prayer of petition to God, reciting it sometimes twice daily and would do so for the next fourteen months.[1]

After the holiday weekend I returned to Philadelphia with the flu. While lying in bed I thought about the times when I was a child and Mom would bring a dinner tray of homemade chicken soup to my bed. I called the memory-care center and told Mom I could not visit her because I was sick, adding, in jest, that I needed her to take care of me. Quickly, she responded in her mothering voice, "You have to learn to take care of yourself and do everything the doctor told you to do." I just cried; I had not heard that mothering voice in such a long time. I was holding on to the past when our roles were not reversed. I remembered the small needlepoint pillow Mom had in her room that read, "A mother's heart is a special place where children always have a home." I never paid too much attention to the pillow but came to understand it from a simple phone call. Home is not a place where your clothes are or a place where you feel safe, but that place for me became a person. Mom was my home. Without her I wondered if I would ever be home again. Whenever I left Mom, my heart lived an orphaned existence.

As I lay in bed sick, listening to her, I did not really want a bowl of her chicken soup; I just wanted her home with me, something I would never have again.

A month later my brother and I took her to the nursing home's annual Christmas party. I dressed Mom in

---

[1] See page 139 for a copy of the prayer.

her finest, fixing her hair and makeup. It was a chance for my brother and me to meet the family members of her housemates. We all shared dinner, and afterward most of them sat listening to the singer but not Mom. Mom loved to dance, and all night she stood on her wobbly knees, standing in one position, swaying with us and dancing for two-plus hours. As long as her family was there, she was happy, and when she was happy, I was happy.

A TENSE BASECAMP

The next day I left New Jersey for my weekly two-hour drive home. How I wished for a warm welcome replete with replenishing hugs and an empathetic ear. Instead I bounced from caring for Mom and battling the enemy to being with my husband, who, I felt, was still angry with me since March 2009, when Mom came to live with us in Houston. In his reality, my absence was a sign of marital and spousal neglect. I was unable to relax my guard or share anything with him about my life. The tension was thick when I walked in the backdoor to the kitchen, dragging my luggage behind me. Paul was cleaning up after dinner.

"Hey, I'm home."

He lashed out a passive response laced with aggressive overtones. "I couldn't think of anything to write in my Christmas letter about you except that you are always with your Mom." I did not have a response to his greeting. All I heard was his anger, and all I could think about was how I hated Christmas letters sent to people who are not in our lives anyway.

While walking past him to the stairs, I once again recalled all the second family dramas when I sat and listened, when he required and received my emotional support over the last twelve years. I went upstairs, refreshed my luggage, and punched my time clock until I "got" to leave again.

My husband had been sick a few weeks prior then began feeling better but decided to stop his antibiotics short of their prescribed course, resulting in a relapse. The following day while he rested in bed until dinnertime, my brother called.

"Hi! I'm in the city."

"Great. Come over for some dinner. Just walk in. I'll unlock the front door. I'll be in the kitchen."

The moment my brother walked in the front door, my husband was coming down the steps for dinner. My brother greeted him, but my husband froze midstep, did not respond, looked at me, and said, "I'm not hungry." He turned around and marched up the steps. My brother, not knowing how he offended him, was now uncomfortable. I told him to watch the stove, and I went upstairs.

"Do you want me to bring dinner up on a tray?"

"No. I didn't want any confusion tonight because I don't feel well."

"What confusion? Mario is just going to sit and eat a meal with us."

"I'll talk to you later. I don't have the energy to talk to you about this right now because I don't feel well."

Inside my mind, my anger raged, *You'll talk to me later?*

I returned to the kitchen to my brother, who asked, "Do you want me to leave?"

"No. He's just having a temper tantrum."

My brother quickly ate his dinner, telling me he felt uncomfortable and wanted to leave immediately. I was so embarrassed and apologized. He told me he understood and left. My heart broke wide open as I felt the unnecessary tension. I cleaned up the kitchen and watched some television—anything to delay going upstairs. When I finally did, as I mounted the steps, I decided this was not the time to vent my anger since he was sick, and I was tired. When I entered the bedroom, he was lying in bed, reading. In silence, I began changing for bed when he broke the silence: "I told you I didn't want any confusion tonight."

Something inside me snapped, and I snapped back, "How dare you make my family feel uncomfortable in our home! Shame on you! All because you decided to stop your antibiotics before their course, everybody has to pay," and off I went into an hour-long rant. I do not remember much else except that I slept upstairs that night. As I climbed the steps, I wished I had had enough energy to pack my suitcase and drive to my brother's house. Mom's needs were my focal point right then, and everyone and everything else was peripheral to me. In my mind nothing was going to stand in my way, and I counted no casualty as too great a loss.

Although I was so appreciative and acutely aware that if it were not for my husband, I would not be able to spend this precious time with Mom, I resented that it came at such a high price. When the enemy was not attacking Mom, I was beginning to experience her unconditional love, but in my marriage the love was, unfortunately, conditional. This blindsided me. I expected him to throw me a lifeline of comfort or tend to my wounds, but it never came. His selfishness just compounded my stress and deep disappointment.

Early the next morning he came upstairs, got under the covers, and, through tears, apologized. We talked for three hours. His apology, laced with the realization of his selfishness, became the catalyst for us attending marriage counseling.

JANUARY 1, 2011– DECEMBER 31, 2011

Sifting Through Memories

It was now April, and I finally felt capable of handling the arduous task of sifting through four floors of memories in my mother's old row home. The two most important chapters in my life were ending at the same time: Mom's life as I knew it and the impending sale of the dwelling that echoed memories spanning 109 years that three generations called home. I found my mother's wedding dress and my grandmother's opera dress, which I donned, fantasizing about their last events. I found my grandmother's family photos, setting them aside for my cousins. I labored over what to keep and what to throw away and what I could and could not let go of...yet. Most days I worked feverishly as a way to keep my emotions at bay, but eventually I would tire and collapse onto the steps in tears.

Mom's house would sell on August 16, 2011. Two days before the sale, I went there to finish cleaning. After I was done, I walked into each room and thanked 1011 for all it was to my family. Saying good-bye was a poignant moment. The next day my brother and I did our final walk through the house while sharing memories of each room. We then buried our keys and our hearts in a hole in the foundation—a foundation that faithfully supported the lives of three generations.

THE ENEMY'S PLAN BACKFIRES

Since Mom's new home was closer to the family beach house and also my brother's residence, it became our daily retreat. Having her home for the day gave me the opportunity to prepare foods she loved. However, instead of Mom commanding her kitchen of thirty years, she just sat on a stool and watched me prepare lunch. I missed her being the woman of the house, making everything from scratch like her mother did. She could no longer cook or remember the recipes once filed in her organized and creative mind. We ate lunch outside then Mom would nap under the umbrella while I gardened. Occasionally she opened her eyes and verbally directed my plantings or smiled, content to know family was near.

Spending the day at my brother's house became our new routine. While there I would make calls to her friends in Philadelphia or to my brother or to her older sister, then ninety, who lived three hours away. I painted her nails, dyed and cut her hair, took her for long wheelchair rides on the boardwalk, or just sat under the pavilion to look out at the water, talk about nature, or joke around. I remember one day sitting with Mom under the pavilion realizing there was nowhere else in the world I would have rather been then right there with her. The purest, most complete, and most intimate love I have ever experienced was with Mom. These were the times when my heart, soul, and emotions were full and at rest. I wondered if this was a byproduct of motherhood. Whatever it was, I wanted to memorize every moment, knowing that every day was a gift and one day God would take her home back to Him.

It was during these times that I began noticing a change. My journal did not reflect a specific incident or date because, many times, changes weave their way into everyday life without permission or recognition. Mom became more playful, not as a result from the disease because she was able to turn it off at will. One day in April while I was gardening, Mom began playing peek-a-boo with her hooded coat, giggling, laughing, and throwing me kisses—something my mother would have never done. A shift was taking place. Something life-changing was happening. A new Mom began to emerge—a Mom that I had never known before but the Mom that I had always longed for.

Photos of Mom before she married showed a very light, fun, and carefree woman, whose stylish apparel matched her gloves, hanky, purse, and hat. However, once she assumed her roles of wife, mother, and caretaking daughter to her parents, she traded in all her style and light-heartedness for an apron and practicality. She became a slave to duty and responsibility, finding her worth through servanthood, where serving became more important than the person she served. Now Mom was finally free from her dutiful role that sabotaged her calling to be her true self. This new Mom contrasted the strict, stoic, and unplayful mother who I remembered and that affected me most. Rarely did she give me attention or affection while growing up. Duty stole her away from me, and my needs, emotional or otherwise, just seemed to interrupt her already too-crowded schedule. Now, even under the enemy's attack, Mom was still evolving emotionally, and God was healing her heart issues, which I knew nothing about.

One night after dinner at the memory-care center, one of the aides came over to Mom to say hello. Surprisingly, Mom pulled her down, held her face in both her hands, and spoke. "I hope all your dreams come true in your life," and she continued giving her words of wisdom and good wishes. The woman's heart was touched, evidenced by the tears welling up in her eyes. Instead of being jealous as I was in the beginning when I learned that Mom wanted to dance with one of the aides, I stood behind her chair in awe, seeing how she freely poured her love out onto others. She still had purpose, and she was still giving and serving, but this time she was serving the purity of her love, overflowing from within.

Another day when Mom was at the cottage, I decided to tie up emotional loose ends in my mother's life. I called her only living brother, then eighty-eight, who had not called or spoken to Mom in about twenty years. He was her youngest brother, who, along with his older brother, had the privilege of attending college, and both became doctors. When the older brother died, he left an inheritance to those siblings who did not have that educational opportunity. Therefore, the younger brother, who had since retired at the age of fifty-two, did not receive an inheritance. During the distribution of the inheritance to the other siblings, this younger brother tried to coerce his remaining siblings into giving him part of their inheritance. Normally, Mom bowed down to everyone else's desires, neglecting her own. I was never quite sure how this episode played out but it fractured the family. His twenty-year snub was punishment for Mom. Over those years she never spoke poorly about or judged him. She always felt bad because growing up they were close, she being the youngest girl and he the youngest boy.

I told Mom it was her brother, and she took the phone from me and asked, with excitement, how he was doing. Awkwardly, they exchanged pleasantries. Sensing a lull in the conversation, I was about to prompt her with another question, but before I could Mom smiled large and said, "I love you." Words that were never spoken in their household or exchanged among siblings left her brother speechless. I just stood next to her, so proud of how she was living unencumbered, overflowing with love to a person who had undeservedly shunned her for being true to herself.

God's love was flowing in her, through her, and out of her to others. The enemy's attacks, purposed to destroy Mom, did not break her down but broke her open. How powerful a moment when a life breaks open like a bottle of perfume, spilling out an aroma of love. The enemy could not touch this intangible and powerful force inside her.

THE ENEMY UNEARTHS GOLD

Not only did Mom begin pouring out her love to others, but she began pouring her love onto me. I began referring to these moments as "golden nuggets." Serendipitously, they would materialize during the routine of our daily lives. I prioritized being with Mom every Wednesday because it was her laundry day. The aides knew not to fold Mom's laundry. This was something she and I did together. It gave her a sense of purpose and accomplishment as it did for me when I was a kid. Mom was a homemaker with a high standard of excellence to the point of ironing her pillowcases and prided herself on how she could fold anything to perfection. Our routine began after preparing her for bed. I put on the television, sat her on the couch, and gave her small towels to fold or colored socks to pair. It took her a while, but she succeeded. I decided to see how she would do if I gave her a shirt. As I stood folding, hoping for victory, she sat struggling, trying to figure out how to join the hanger to the shirt. Defeated and upset with herself, she collapsed her arms, her head, the shirt, the hanger and her confidence. "I used to be able to do this; now I can't."

I shut off the TV, knelt in front of her, held her face in my hands, and said, "Mom, we don't love you for what you do; we love you for who you are." My statement was a revelation to her because Mom believed people loved her only for all the service she provided.

A smile beamed across her face. "Thank you. No one ever told me that."

We hugged for a long time—another golden-nugget moment with Mom that healed her heart and mine. That night when I put Mom to bed, I knelt next to the bed like I always did and laid my head next to hers for pillow talk. That night I told her I loved her, and she said she loved me too. Her words sat on my heart like a missing piece to a puzzle sealed in a golden moment.

Another unexpected golden nugget was unearthed while sitting Mom on the edge of the bed to apply lotion to her feet. With all lucidity, Mom broke the silence: "I know I'm nuts. I know I'm not on the right train, and I hope it's not interfering with your life."

Through tears, I barely eked out, "No, Mom, you are not interfering with my life. You are the biggest part of my life."

Then from a gentle, honest, open, and sweet place, she expressed to me, in her own way, how much she loved me.

"You and I live in our own little world. We are like two cells on the globe, and God loves us. You are the only one who understands me, and I could always depend on you. I hit the jackpot having you as a daughter."

Words that I thirsted to hear my whole life flowed from her lips with ease. Within this realm of intimacy, our relationship continued to heal. I lived for intimate moments with Mom, moments we never had before, moments when her words filled up my love tank and imprinted her love DNA into my soul. Although this horrible disease was taking my mother from me ever so slowly, it was giving her to me for the first time. She had become my best friend, and I had become hers. We not only loved one another, but we finally liked and fully accepted one another. I had crawled into her soul, and she had crawled into mine. We had become one another's soul mates because we helped one another's souls grow to a place they never could have without the other's influence.

The next morning Mom and I sat on the couch enjoying the warm sunshine streaming in through the window. Mom did my favorite thing. She held my face in her hands, placed her nose right up to mine, looked straight into my eyes, and while tapping her forefinger on my face, said, "I

wish for you to be as happy as you are right now—always."
In my heart I knew my happiness would never be as full as
it was in that moment. It was full because she was there.

Wondering what other golden nuggets were inside
her that I had not already mined led me to ask Mom questions. While doing her hair one morning I asked, "Mom,
do you remember the first time Daddy kissed you?"

Quickly she responded, "Yes, I do. It was wonderful
because I knew it wouldn't be the last." Her response not
only surprised me because that was a sound thought for
someone battling Alzheimer's.

Another time I asked what she would change about
herself if she had anything to change. Immediately she
responded, "To be beautiful."

In my eyes she was more beautiful than ever, although
she could never comprehend my thought. Mom never
had a high opinion of herself. One day a few of the aides
saw her in the hallway and made a fuss over her. As we
walked past them, I told Mom how many people loved
her, adding, "There is only one person who doesn't love
you, and that person is you."

Surprisingly she agreed. "You are right. People only
like me when I'm doing for them. I've always felt that way,
and I've always felt like I was doing the wrong thing."

Her response told me that the enemy had been whispering into her ear years before her incarceration. I now
understood why Mom was so emphatic, vigilant, and cautious about doing the right thing. My mother was finally
sharing her deepest thoughts with me, and for the first
time in my life, I felt like I was getting to know her as a
woman and not just as my mother—a monumental feat
for any daughter.

One day I arrived at Mom's memory-care home. She was in her wheelchair, asleep in the activities room, so I knelt next to her and kissed her awake. She opened her eyes, smiled, grabbed my face, and kissed me so softly as if I had become part of her interrupted dream. We hugged, kissed, and snuggled for a long time while others watched our love fest. I knew people judged Mom and me as we interacted. They did not understand our blatant affection for each other; however, I did not care because we were making up for lost time. With God's help she and I had been working on something profoundly important to our souls. What they were seeing was our jubilation over the goldmine that God had unearthed between us. I felt sorry for them because I think everyone in life should experience this level of joy and intimacy. Back in her room, we sat on the couch, and she said, "Thank you for including me into your life."

"Thank you for including me in yours, Mom."

We hugged, snuggled, and wrestled until dinner. Mom was the only old woman I knew who loved to wrestle. That night when I put her to bed, she thanked me for being her daughter, and I thanked her for being my Mom. The love between us was now unbridled, and our hearts were soaring.

However, my favorite golden-nugget memory happened while shopping to replace her broken glasses. While waiting for the clerk, I began trying eyeglasses on Mom. As I knelt in front of her wheelchair evaluating the size, fit, style, and shape of the glasses, Mom grabbed my face with her both hands and joyfully exclaimed, "I would never have believed that I would have had a daughter like you, so beautiful, so on top of everything, and you are mine!"

"You are mine, too, Mom. Mom, out of the millions of mothers God could have given me, He gave me you, and out of the millions of daughters He could have given you, He gave you me. Mom, we had a divine appointment!" She smiled so big, and we kissed and hugged, engulfed in a joy bubble. Time froze for us to have a deep, intimate moment in an eyeglass store as if no one around us existed. Mom and I found the richness of every moment and lived that moment to the fullest. After that I tried every pair of goofy glasses on Mom and myself and took pictures while laughing at one another. It reminded me of our shopping trips to the department stores when I was a kid. Whenever I would pass by the hat display, I would pick out the silliest hat and put it on to get her to laugh, which became our shopping ritual and the rare time when I could joke with her.

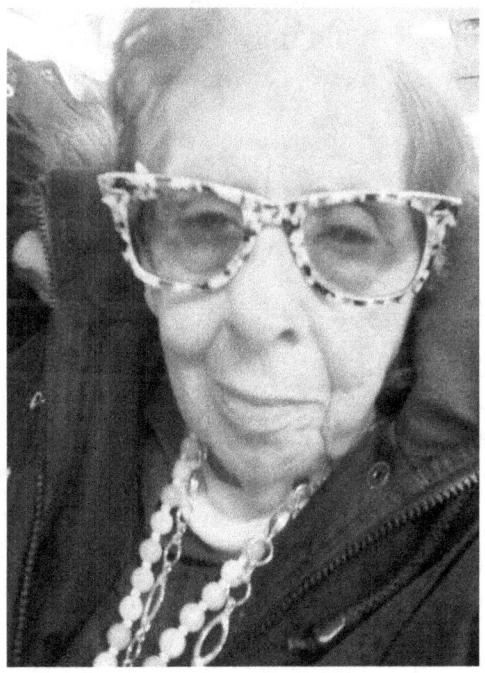

Mom, showing her great sense of humor by wearing the goofiest eyeglasses I could find in the store.

I could never define what I needed from Mom, but I did know there was something I desperately needed. In these golden-nugget moments, she was unknowingly giving me that indeterminate, yet essential, ingredient that my daughter/soul needed. I truly believe that as I supplanted her mother, I was giving her what her daughter/soul missed from her duty-bound mother. As daughters, both of our souls were healing deeply from these golden-nugget moments.

I continued praying my daily prayer over Mom, knowing He is a faithful God. I believed I would see His resurrection power amid this horrible situation because God never wastes the pain and sorrows woven into our circumstances. I knew I would see a resurrection because resurrection always follows a sacrifice of love, and this was its beginning.

REALIZING MY SECRET WEAPON

It was during these golden-nugget moments that my understanding began to crystallize concerning the answer to God's test question set before me years earlier: How will you respond to the adversity the enemy is aiming at you? It was a love test, and the answer is one word: love. I was to respond with love because love is the most powerful force on earth and defeats anything in the enemy's arsenal. God's goal was to strengthen me for my sojourn here on earth in both character and heart. I was asking Him to remove the mountain, but instead He would take me through it and change my heart by it. I was asking God to get me out of this situation, but God wanted me to ask, "What can I get out of this situation?" I was concerned about what was happening to me, but God was more concerned about what was happening in me. I had given God all the brokenness of this situation, knowing that nothing is ever wasted in His economy. The enemy's goal was to destroy. God's goal was to rebuild, save, and replenish.

There was no question that the enemy was a wise and calculating foe, but there was a breach in his plan. He developed his strategies by targeting my weakness—my deep love for my mother—but failed to recognize my greatest strength—my deep love for my mother. The day I realized that love was my greatest weapon was the day my perspective shifted, and I silently declared war. Love was now the armor I wore and the momentum that propelled me forward. I was now the militant launching preemptive love attacks against the enemy's now-fruitless attempts. My new position was offensive and my resolve tenacious as steel. Love was now my battle cry.

AMBUSHED IN THE HALLWAY

One dark, rainy morning I arrived at the home before breakfast to a symphony of activity. Nurses were administering medications. Aides were administering morning care. Others were seating the residents in the activities room to watch the news until breakfast was served, but I could not find Mom anywhere. I asked one of the aides, "Where's my mom?"

"She didn't want to be in the activities room with the others; she wanted to be placed in the hallway."

I checked the hallways and still could not find her.

"What hallway?"

"The one down at the end."

I found the hallway I never knew existed; it was located far from everyone. I stood at the top of the long corridor and saw Mom at the other end sitting on her walker, hunched over a small cup of water, staring through the large glass door out at the dark, rainy morning. Mom had separated herself from others, as she always did. I stood there for a minute watching her as tears welled up in my eyes, knowing she felt discarded and unloved by my brother and me for placing her there. Easily recognizing the enemy's retreating strategy, I was not going to allow him victory over Mom or me anymore. Standing there, I recalled a sermon I had heard about not holding on to people too tightly, that we are all on loan to one another, and ultimately we all belong to God. I realized that she was God's daughter long before she was my mother and began viewing this situation as part of her soul's journey and that ultimately God was in control and loved her more than I ever could. Taking another long moment to compose myself, I approached her, knelt down, and in an upbeat voice asked, "Hey, Mom, whatcha doing?"

She gave me a sideways glance but continued looking forward, forcing a response. "What time did you get up? What are you doing here?"

"Mom, I'm here to spend the day with you."

She kept staring at the darkness outside the door. Intuitively, I knew Mom was taking inventory of her life as she always did, feeling cast aside and powerless with no voice to veto our decision. With my new love weaponry, I took her into her room and began fixing her hair before breakfast, but she remained distant and quiet. During breakfast she was verbally combative toward me, but I was patient and did not stop loving her through service. Afterward I took her back to her room to brush and floss her teeth, remaining steadfast, knowing my love could outlast the onslaught of the enemy. Finally, she began sharing how sad she was at how her life had turned out and how much she missed my dad—something that she would never have shared with me in our past relationship. I sat her on the couch, pulled a large box out of the closet that I took from her Philadelphia home, sat next to her, and began reading her my father's cards and love letters from the beginning of their courtship. She, of course, forgot that she saved every card from every occasion over the years. As I read them to her, her smile grew large. "Did he write that to me?" She then made herself comfortable and read each one herself.

A day that began poorly with an attack was neutralized by the love of a man who now expressed his love from the grave.

SIMPLE LOVE

I learned that loving someone does not have to be complicated or largely demonstrated. I found that the simplest things brought joy into her life and recognized that love is in the details. When I was growing up, Mom never left the house without applying lipstick. This became our new ritual before leaving her room. I would apply lipstick onto myself then onto her bottom lip for her to smudge her lips together to apply it to her top lip. However, over time she was unable to do this anymore, so I began applying another layer to my lips and kissed her dead center onto her lips, and she said, "Now that's the way to apply lipstick!" Her mood elevated, and she felt loved. To this day I cannot apply lipstick without thinking of Mom.

The memory-care facility would have weekly live performances for the residents. At this one particular event, they handed out long, brightly colored necklaces. Mom, a woman who wore an occasional nondescript necklace to work, was captivated by them and would not take them off even for bed. Again, another surprising and repressed part of Mom began to emerge. Looking for necklaces together became a favorite shopping outing, resulting in about a thirty-plus necklace collection. Even my friends bought her necklaces, adding to her collection. One of the first things I did when arriving for a visit was to pick out three or four necklaces to coordinate with her outfit or pajamas. I recall one time putting the necklaces on her, and she grabbed my face and kissed it all over while telling me how I made her day, month, and year. She proudly wore them during the day, showing them to people wherever I took her and awaiting their praise. I was so thrilled when I discovered something so small that made her so happy.

Anything I could do or find that brought her joy I exploited to the hilt because I knew I was outmaneuvering the enemy. I made something as simple as a shower into a spa experience. Unlike the five-minute showers the aides gave her during the week, I would leave her to sit while the hot water caressed her tired body, and she would ooze, "Ohhhhh, this feels soooo good!"

Every few minutes I would peek inside the shower curtain. "Mom, are you doing okay?"

With closed eyes she would respond, "I'm great. This feels sooooo good!" I loved watching her luxuriate under the hot water. I took boring rituals and turned them into fun as any mother would do for her child. I even made up a song that I would sing each night while she brushed her teeth, and we would dance to it.

When I finally got her dressed, we would sit on the couch together and talk until she fell asleep nestled into my chest. Every now and then she would awake and ask me if I locked the front door, thinking we were at 1011 in Philadelphia. After putting her to bed, I would kneel on the floor for pillow-talk time, and we would tell each other how much we loved one another. One night during pillow talk, she began talking about all her family, asking me who was alive and who was dead. After inventorying everyone's death status, Mom replied, "Now they are waiting for me." We then prayed together. Believing we were home, she would shuffle her body to the edge of the bed asking, "Do you have enough room?"

"Mom, I'm going to stay up and watch TV. I'll be in later."

"Oh, okay. Don't stay up too late."

I would watch TV until her meds kicked in then pray my prayer over her. Some nights I would leave; other nights I would just sit in the dark while she slept, relishing the peace-filled silence.

WAR COUNCIL

One morning while I was walking in the main entrance, the head nurse summoned me into her office to talk about

Mom. I felt like a soldier attending a war council to receive an update on the enemy's advancing techniques. Mom was exhibiting signs of aggression in the morning, and they wanted to administer the lowest dose of an antianxiety medication at 6:00 a.m. to shower her because she was "assaulting" the aides during morning care—biting them, pulling their hair, and the like. As she spoke, my mind stayed on the word "assaulting." I thought "assaulting" was a glaringly criminal word to use mainly because I associated this word with premeditation. In the theater of my mind, the enemy was the bully assaulting my mother, and, through her, he was the one assaulting the aides. Once again his cowardly and covert antics made Mom culpable, keeping himself blameless. Failing at keeping my mind on the conversation, I wondered what word described an enemy using someone to commit a war crime. As she spoke, I wished she had delivered this message with a more compassionate tone. When I first met her, she told me that her mother had died from Alzheimer's disease. However, the empathy she once felt seemed to have faded into business jargon. It saddened me that that she had not experienced Mom's love and giving nature. When I snapped back to the sound of her voice, feeling like I was being reprimanded for Mom's behavior caused by her illness, I softly asked the obvious.

"Is Mom the only one who is aggressive like this?"

"No."

"Oh."

My rhetorical question magnified her condemning tone, and she softened. I never knew how to respond except to say, "I'm really sorry." I dreaded these invitations and was happy when they were over and the issues resolved. I now understood how mothers felt when summoned into the principal's office for their child's poor behavior.

Yes, these verbal reports meant Alzheimer's was advancing, but in my mind it did not matter anymore because Mom and I had already defeated him. All his plans were now futile. No matter what he did, he could not take away the fact that he had given me the mother I had always longed for and gave Mom the daughter she had hoped for and envisioned. I left her office and hurried to see my mother. Now, instead of the ninety-foot-long hallway being something I despised, I joyfully sped through it to get to Mom; even if she was having a bad day, I knew love would make it a great day.

LAUGHTER AS A WEAPON

Over time an unexpected weapon in my love arsenal began to emerge: laughter. As the enemy broke Mom open, he unearthed another part of her personality I never knew existed—an amazing sense of humor. Mom began making me laugh as I had never laughed before, and I saw Mom laugh so hard from the depths of her soul as I had never seen her laugh before. Sharing intense times of laughter brought deep healing to our relationship. Now when the enemy used his tactics to confuse her, it became the catalyst for her and me to laugh—not at her but at the enemy. Laughter washed away our sadness, rendering his weaponry ineffective. Like two eagles, we now soared above the storm.

Early one morning I received a call from Mom's nurse telling me that the night before, while leaving the room after administering my mother's meds, Mom had fallen out of bed and gotten hurt. I left home immediately.

When I arrived, I found her napping in her wheelchair in the activities room. I knelt next to her, seeing her black and blue hand, wrist, and eye. After kissing her awake, I asked, "Mom, what happened to your hand?"

Never wanting to draw attention to herself, she slowly sat up, lifted her arm and began turning her hand and wrist as if seeing them for the first time. After thoroughly examining her black and blue hand, she looked at me and said, "You should have seen the other guy." Her response told me that she did not want me to worry and that she was okay. Indirectly, she was taking care of me. After telling my friend Barbara this story, she commented on how amazed she was that this disease did not touch Mom's sense of humor. It was intact, quick, and sharp—another part of Mom's personality the enemy couldn't touch.

Later that morning I took her to the cottage for the day. After lunch I brought her into the bathroom. As I began washing her "PP," as we called it, Mom, looking down at my handiwork, softly inquired, "Do you do this for all your company?" I began living my life between the intense satisfaction of tender-filled, intimate moments and extreme laughter. "No, Mom, I just do this for you because 'you special cus-ta-ma'!"

When Mom shopped at the outdoor Italian market a block from her Philadelphia home, her favorite Chinese vendor would always say to her after giving her the price, "You special cus-ta-ma!" Over the years we adopted this as part of our family lingo.

My friend Barbara had dinner with us one evening at my brother's home. Afterward Mom looked at us and asked, "Where's Mac?" meaning my father. I gently said, "Mom, he's dead." She looked perplexed and asked, "Then who did I break up with last week?" Barb and I could not stop laughing. Mom laughed too. These were the times when I experienced her as a girl in her twenties who dated and broke up with boys.

Whenever I picked her up or took her home, we had to pass by a jewelry store called Corinne Jewelers. Each time her unusual name would be flashing on the neon sign: "Corinne, Corinne, Corinne." I would always make a big fuss, and she would smile from ear to ear to see her name flashing in lights, not remembering we saw it earlier that day. One day we were stopped at a red light in front of the sign. As usual, like a mother making her child aware of a cow on the side of the road, I said, "Mom, look, Corinne Jewelers!"

However, this time she did not respond with her usual excitement but looked perplexed, turned to me, and asked, "Do I own a jewelry store?" The light turned green, and horns honked behind me, but I was unable to drive because I was laughing so hard.

After spending a day at the cottage, I readied Mom to take her to the home early because every Thursday they had live performances for the memory-care and assisted-living residents. These were some of my favorite times with Mom as she sang along or clapped her hands and bounced her legs to the beat. That afternoon when I told her it was time to go, Mom, believing it was Sunday, asked, "Are we going to church?"

"No, Mom, I'm taking you to a singing show."

I put her into the car, and for some reason going to church became going to a funeral. For the next fifteen minutes we had the same cyclical conversation.

"Are we going to a funeral?"

"No, Mom, we're not going to a funeral."

Until she finally let it go. Having repetitive and exhausting conversations was one of the enemy's tactics to wear down my kindness and lash out with impatience, attacking the one I loved. Driving in silence was a welcomed reprieve.

After wheeling Mom through the front door of the memory-care home, I realized it was St. Patrick's Day and was happy to see such a festive atmosphere. The place was packed with about a hundred or so people. They were handing out drinks, hor d'oeuvres, colored necklaces, and balloons. Family members accompanied their loved ones to the Thursday events. Many were taking photos of the entertainers for the day, a husband-and-wife team who were in their late sixties to early seventies.

The well-endowed woman had on high heels and a short, tight black dress with an overflowing and plunging neckline, topped with a flamboyant floor-length electric-green cape trimmed in lime-green boa feathers. Her husband donned a green leprechaun's outfit with thick green sparkly suspenders and a long green wig topped off with a tall green sparkly leprechaun's hat. Like a mother whose child was seeing a Disney character for the first time, I stooped down next to Mom. "Mom, what do you think of all this?"

Her forehead lined with confusion, she leaned forward in her chair, twisting her body to look at me, and said, "I've never been to a funeral like this before."

I literally buckled over with laughter. During the entire show she thought she was at a funeral, forbidding me to clap because that is not proper behavior at a funeral and disrespectful to the person whose dead body lay in front.

That night while putting her to bed, she thanked me for being her daughter and told me when she was pregnant with me that she prayed to God for a good daughter. She then she told me to love God and love my parents and for Mario and me to love one another. I wished I could have put her to bed every night for moments like those.

DOCTOR VISITS

My mother was a people watcher, so taking Mom to the doctor was always an adventure. While sitting in the office, I would attempt to read a magazine while keeping my eye on her. Inevitably an overweight person would walk by. I would close my eyes, hoping she would not say it, but I knew it was coming. She would lean sideways toward me; I called it "the Corinne lean." Because her hearing was not good, her whispers were louder than her normal voice.

"He didn't miss too many meals."

"Mom, shhhh!"

"What? I'm just making an observation. Don't you think he's fat??"

I could not help but laugh like a mother observing her child's innocent, truthful, yet unsuitable comment. Most Alzheimer's doctors would have labeled that inappropriate behavior, but I knew it was just Mom living her life out loud. She would have said that to me with or without the disease but in a lower tone.

When I had to go to the bathroom, I would tell Mom I would be right back. Thankfully she was always good in the doctor's office. However, as I began walking towards the facility Mom would shout in front of everyone "mention my name, they'll give you a good seat." Her sense of humor was always on point and warmed my heart like nothing else could.

The foot doctor always had a crowded waiting room. My mother was a patient woman but since this disease, had the patience of a gnat. To manage her impatience, I would grab a magazine from the crowded rack and hand it to her, hoping to restrain her impatience and commentary about everyone. Mom loved reading signs on the street or highlighted boxes in magazines. As I refocused my eyes on my magazine, she read, in one of her loud whispers, the large sideline on the front of the woman's magazine for all to hear.

"Twelve sex positions to pleasure your mate."

"Mom, give me the magazine!"

"Why? You just gave it to me. What's wrong? Am I hurting anybody?"

She would never let it go but just kept the conversation going. Like a mother, I did not know whether to laugh or correct her.

The doctor was finally available to see us. He walked in with seven other resident/student associates. After he had introduced himself, Mom read aloud and commented on his Italian name embroidered across his lab coat. He was not only Italian and a doctor but extremely handsome—a trifecta in her eyes. Mom turned on the charm and began trying to fix me up with him. Hoping to derail her match-making efforts, I softly stated, "Mom, I'm married."

"You are? This is the first time I'm hearing about this! When were you going to tell me?"

Round and round we went in front of the doctor and his associates, who were looking at us as if we had ten heads. On the way out of his office, her favorite thing to do was fill her pockets with as many candies from the candy dish as her hands could accommodate while telling the receptionist that she loved me "with cosmetics and without cosmetics" and waving good-bye as she sang and danced her way out the door. My once-quiet and reserved mother was now the life of the party even when there was no party. This is when I loved her to pieces, and the enemy couldn't touch us. Although he had Mom incarcerated, she no longer lived like a prisoner.

Another time at the beach house, we were sitting on the couch, and I hugged her and told her I loved her, and softly she responded, "I love you too. Why else would I put up with your crap?"

I pulled away from our embrace, seeing her grinning ear to ear, knowing she got me. I had found the eye of the storm: Mom's loving intimacy along with laughter. Truly, I have never laughed so hard in my life at the character she always was but never displayed.

MOVING AGAIN

For the past two years, I had been driving weekly to New Jersey for my three day visit and was beyond exhausted. I spoke to my husband, and we decided to move closer to Mom. We put our house in Philadelphia on the market in September, and although we only lived there for a little over one year, the house sold in ten days with competing bids over comps amid a bad economy. We offered a bid on a home in New Jersey that was not even on the market and it was accepted. It was a God thing! I was thrilled to leave Philadelphia's pain-filled memories and reduce my stress levels and long commute.

During the mornings I set up our new home, and in the afternoons and evenings I cared for Mom. One night during pillow-talk time, she asked, "How much longer will we have together?" Tears welled up in my eyes because I could not imagine life without her. It was a question tired and elderly people ask themselves. There comes a time when they instinctively know that their time is near.

"I don't know, Mom, but what I do know is that we will spend eternity together."

It was December 16, 2011. We took Mom to the home's annual Christmas party, where she still got up and danced but not with as much energy or passion as the last year. Christmastime had always been a busy time for Mom, especially Christmas Eve, Mom's yearly shining moment when she carried on traditions passed down from her mother, turning out a traditional Italian seven-course fish dinner to a crowd of twenty. This, too, was now all gone from her list of duties. My brother and I now made her the seven fish, and like many of her guests over the years, she was now able to just show up and enjoy the meal and be served.

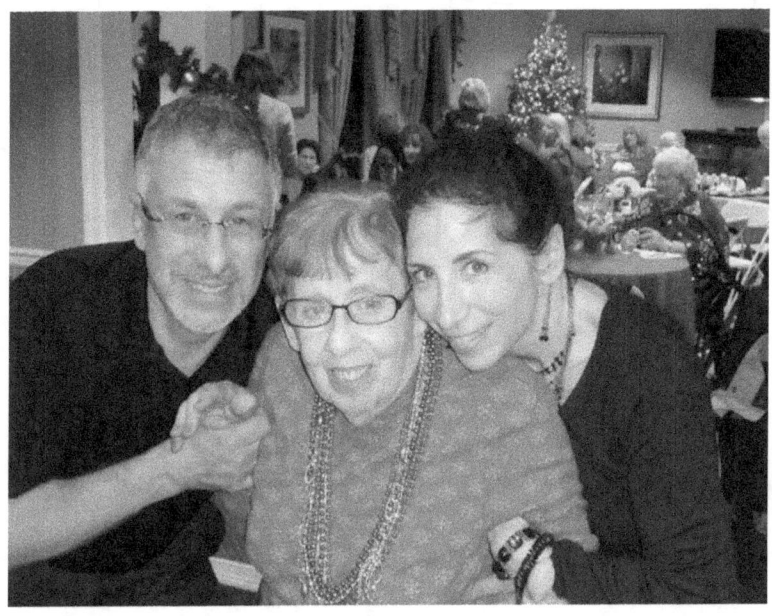

After dancing at the Christmas party two months before her death, my brother and I hold Mom up for a photo op.

JANUARY 1, 2012–
FEBRUARY 12, 2012

THE SILENT ASSASSIN

The enemy no longer warred with me through Mom in hand-to-hand combat, verbal abuses, or surprise attacks. Instead he now took his military maneuvers underground, deep inside her brain. His power, however, could only reach her physical brain and not the treasures of her heart, soul, or spirit – the true essence of her being.

The first signs of the enemy's undercover work were Mom's inability to use a spoon or direct food into her mouth. She fluctuated between eating half of what she normally ate to eating very little. Like with a six-month-old baby, I now spoonfed my mother-child. However, unlike a new mother, I followed it by massaging her throat to facilitate swallowing. When that failed, I ended up clearing her mouth of food squirreled away in her cheeks. Some days she ate and swallowed. Other days it took me hours to feed her one small pudding, and water dribbled out of her mouth as quickly as I put it in. When she would not eat a banana or a dessert, her favorites, I knew the end was near. Her weight dropped from 132 to 117 and was falling because she was eating less and less. Her appetite for this world and all it had to offer was diminishing. Outings were no longer part of our routine. She was now content sitting in her room on the couch with her head nestled into my chest.

DEMOBILIZING

When the home recommended a hospital bed for her room, my heart skipped a beat. My mind flashed back to our first tour of the residents' rooms. Immediately, I noticed the healthier residents' rooms were decorated with homey touches. However, the rooms of those whose health was beginning to fail were slowly stripped of their homey décor, which was replaced with hospital beds, trays, and oxygen tanks. I decorated Mom's room to be a scaled-down version of her former home, 1011, but now the room decorated with such care and comfort was being dismantled to make room for the hospital bed and rolling trays.

Mom did not want to stand anymore, fearing another fall so the home got her a "geri chair." This was a chair in which she could freely recline as they wheeled her. As Mom continued to shut down, I was told I could no longer shower her because it was too difficult and dangerous. Our spa moments had ended. While I was bathing her in bed, she told me not to do something, but I knew I had to do it for her to be clean. After fifty-three years of trying, with a defeated and disgusted voice, she finally conceded, "I can't change you."

Tears welled up in my eyes, quelling my sudden revelation that I thought but could not utter: *Mom, you already did.*

After dressing her for bed in her red and white night-gown, I took out red beads and white pearl necklaces and placed them around her neck. She exhibited so much joy and excitement and, with a big smile, grabbed my face and kissed me softly. It brought tears to my eyes seeing Mom as a sweet old woman. After adorning her with jewels, I applied red lipstick on us both for a photo op. She tried to goof around with me as we always did, but she lacked the energy to do so. Her intent, however, was there, and I knew that although the enemy was making inroads, she was still in there.

Mom's ability to communicate was slowly declining. As her emotional age descended, I adjusted the way I addressed her and now spoke as a mother would speak to her toddler. To define our relationship I would say, "I love my mommy," and she would respond, "I love my daugh-ter." Now she uttered the words through slurring lips. These words were the last ones she spoke to me. Maybe they were the first words she ever spoke to me when I was the age she now reflected. I'll never know.

Mom and I continued living in our insulated world even though everything was unraveling around us with great speed. My brother called to tell me he was going to make funeral arrangements. Intellectually, I knew this was the appropriate thing to do, but emotionally it upset me because it seemed cold and unloving while making her departure a reality. Then, two weeks later, Mom's nurse, Jean, called to tell me they were taking her off all her medications. My heart skipped another beat. Time was collapsing in on her, and God was slowing pulling her back to Him.

Hospice Care

The home called in hospice care, and I met with the representative who introduced me to this unbelievable organization of angels. I could tell that none of these men and women worked at the job to make a living. Their work was a higher calling to make a difference in people's lives. Although their office is the bedside of your loved one, and their coworker was death, their attitudes were for the living.

The first woman I met, Jore, entered Mom's room at eight-thirty at night. After introductions, she proudly announced her résumé. "I've had the privilege of transitioning over one hundred souls. It has been an honor." When I asked about her personal past, she revealed little except to say, "I took a large pay cut, but I am richer now than I've ever been." She told me that many under her care talk to their relatives on the other side, explaining, "They are living between two worlds." She then shared a story about a woman near death who loved Frank Sinatra's music. Jore got herself a long cane, a top hat, and some Sinatra tapes. Donned in her formal apparel, in front of the hospital bed in a nursing home, she sang and performed every song with dancing leg kicks. "I didn't care what anyone thought because I was performing for an audience of one," she exclaimed. Sharing her joy-filled experiences and view of death brought me peace because I knew also, by my faith, that death is not the end. It is just a new beginning.

While hospice care was there, I met about five women and one man, each telling one amazing story after another of their joy-filled experiences accompanying others toward death. They became an extension of me esteeming Mom, knowing that serving her or any other person at this time was a privilege.

One day a new hospice nurse came into Mom's room with a beaming smile, full of enthusiasm. Tracey hugged Mom and me as if we were longtime friends. Tracey seemed a bit different from the others.

Since Mom never wanted to go gray, I held up a box of hair dye, and asked Tracey if she would help me dye Mom's hair. Her smile, now intermingled with a mischievous look, beamed as she walked toward the door and locked it. While holding the doorknob, she looked over her shoulder and proudly whispered, "I know how to dye a person's hair in bed." Everything was an exciting event for her. Mom studied our conversation, and I wondered if she understood what I was asking of Tracey. I mixed the hair dye and applied it to Mom's tired, flopping head. After ten minutes, Tracey placed a heavy-duty trash bag on the edge of the bed. Like those of an infant, Mom's eyes were wide open, and her appearance was thin and fragile. I felt like a new mother being taught how to care for my newborn by a more experienced woman. Mom's eyes studied us as we carefully maneuvered her shoulders and head onto the trash bag. Mom moaned desperately, searching for her voice to yell at me the question she always asked in my youth: "What the hell are you doing?"

With Tracey's infectious smile and excitement, I responded, "Mom, we're dyeing your hair!" As I cradled her in my arms, she relaxed into this unusual spa experience as Tracey, with a rag and a pan of water, slowly and methodically squeezed the warm water onto her scalp, removing the dye. While holding her in position, I realized that I did not escape one part of motherhood. I was experiencing motherhood backward. Instead of birthing an infant, taking her from cradle through childhood to adulthood and releasing her with joy, I birthed an adult, taking her from rebellious teenager back through childhood to cradle to infancy and soon to her death to be reborn into her new life in heaven.

After blow drying her hair, I took a picture of Mom with Tracey even though Mom threw her hand up in front of her face as she always did. However, we held it down for a photo op. I knew I was going against her lifelong wish not to be photographed, but I was being selfish, knowing that this was the last time I would do her hair. I wanted to catalog her last days just like a new mother catalogs the first days of her newborn.

With each day Mom looked more and more like a rigid and frightened newborn. By the next morning Mom moaned to communicate her discomfort. Each new and descending stage of motherhood left me as a novice, so I was relieved when Tracey arrived, took control, and told me what was wrong. "She needs her diaper changed."

I offered to help Tracey and began removing Mom's diaper. Since gentleness has never been my strong suit, I pulled the diaper. Tracey was quick to correct me. "No, don't do it that way. You can break her skin." I recoiled, watched, and learned the ways in which she moved with gentle efficiency. We then began washing Mom, whose eyes were now closed. Tracey talked and talked about how she loved her job and caring for those who could not care for themselves. She talked about her wonderful experiences ushering people toward death. I was happy to meet and be around people who had the same attitude toward death as I did.

In a moment of silence, the squeezing of the sponge made its crackling noise against the bedpan. Tracey stopped for a second. Her smile and eyes grew larger and brighter. "Mom might pass while we are washing her because it is such a nurturing experience." I froze for a second as I was not ready for that to happen, but Tracey continued in her excitement, "How great to have her daughter washing her while she dies."

I just loved her perspective. "Yes, I love caring for Mom. It has been my highest privilege."

She never stopped talking. I was happy to hear all about her life and experiences. After we finished, I realized that she had made washing Mom into a ceremony.

It was now Tuesday, February 7, and I received a call that Mom was now on oxygen and morphine. Knowing her death was near, I packed my bags for an extended stay and rushed to the home to be with her. I was with her this entire journey and did not want her to be alone or with strangers when her soul and spirit left her body. I wanted her to see family by her side and that she was not forsaken but loved to the end.

For the next five nights, I would lay on the couch wide awake, listening to the rhythmic oxygen machine while checking on Mom periodically. Every two hours throughout those nights, one of her aides would arrive, and together we would reposition Mom in the bed. At 2:00 a.m., Nicole turned on the bathroom light. In its glow, we positioned ourselves on either side of Mom and grabbed the sheet under her to roll her over gently. As Nicole stood on one side and I on the other, I looked over at Nicole with tears in my eyes at seeing Mom this incapacitated. As we began moving her, Mom began moaning. Nicole finally said, "Stop. I won't do this to her," believing that moving her was causing Mom pain. However, knowing Mom as well as I did, I sensed she was moaning because she never liked being moved in the dark in her bed, unaware of its edge. Whatever the reason, I was happy that the moaning stopped.

After Nicole left, I watched Mom sleep, wishing I could sleep that deeply. It was the type of rest that declared, "I have no energy left for anyone or anything." She had lived, moved, and served for the past eighty-three years. She was done. Her time was near.

By the following day, an unconscious Mom lay tilted onto her left shoulder with her eyes closed. I did her nails for the last time, knowing I was preparing her, like an undertaker's beautician, for her viewing. The room was quiet except for the pulsating oxygen tank. I took her hand, which was slowly turning blue, and began applying her favorite shade of hot pink. I announced aloud to the enemy that pink and blue were Mom's favorite colors, so even though his goal was death, it had no sting. Believing she could still hear me in her unconscious state, I continued to joke with her as I always did about my constant complaint. "Finally, Mom, you're staying still during a manicure."

Later that morning Tracey arrived with her effervescent smile and announced, "It's time to change the bed linens." I followed her instructions as we gently moved my unconscious mother from one side of the bed to the other, and, like magic, the bed was changed under her to perfection. Being a quintessential homemaker, Mom would have loved the efficiency, work ethic, and joy-filled servant that Tracey embodied.

MOTHERHOOD

My brother's longtime friend John came to see Mom. He had lost his mother years earlier, and this rekindled his emotions. He stood by her bed, bowed his head, and prayed. His emotions for his mother overflowed at Mom's bedside. As he turned around, the tears on his cheeks touched my heart so deeply. There is nothing comparable to the mysterious, undeniable, and far-reaching arm of a mother's love. For many, like me, it is the supremacy of all human love. Even the Bible records the words of Jesus, Who, while hanging on the cross in excruciating pain, made special provision for His mother.

> *When Jesus saw his mother standing there beside the disciple he loved, he said to her, "Dear woman, here is your son." And he said to this disciple, "Here is your mother." And from then on this disciple took her into his home. John 19:26-27 NLT.*

Throughout my entire journey with Mom, the premise of motherhood occupied my thoughts as she moved through descending growth stages. I marveled at the entire phenomenon of motherhood probably because I never was one. A mother's womb is God's workroom, where He forms His mysteries in secret. Moreover, from this secret workroom another person grows inside, and then he or she emerges out of that person. If God, the Creator of life, had not designed it to be such an intrinsic part of nature, it could be a page from a sci-fi novel. Who else but God could have designed such a unique and intimate relationship? He also tells us that every child is so special to Him that He knew each one before any of us are even formed in our mothers' wombs (Jeremiah 1:5). This person was my lifeline during my incubation and the first person who loved me while I was forming. We were hand chosen by God to belong to one another. To me, this relationship was sacred not only because of the miracle that took place in her womb but because it was the only person in the whole world who held and could hold that position in my life.

BIRTHING POSITION

Mom was now lying in her bed in a fetal position, and as well as I knew her body, she now looked to be about eighty-five pounds. Her nurse from the home, Jean, arrived. After administering morphine, Jean rolled up two dry washcloths, pried open Mom's hands, and placed them in as Mom's hand recoiled around them. Having pried open her hands all day to prevent her nails from digging into her skin, I asked Jean, "Why does Mom do that? I keep trying to open her hands, but they keep closing into a fist."

Jean responded, "Many people curl up into the fetal position and close their hands into a fist. I believe they are getting into the fetal position to be birthed into the next realm. These days prior to death are labor pains."

Her thought was so beautiful and paralleled my personal thoughts of reverse motherhood.

When I saw Tracey later that day, I shared this thought with her. Tracey smiled large, as she always did, and said, "Oh, yes. I see it all the time, and I agree. It's a beautiful thing to watch someone transition to the next world."

I realized I was ushering my infant child back toward birth into another realm. I viewed Mom's bed as a womb and the cable from her oxygen mask as the umbilical cord. Her eyes, sometimes a quarter opened but mostly shut, resembled those of a floating fetus in the womb.

Day after day Mom just lay there in a coma. Rarely did I ever see my mother relax. She was in constant motion, enslaved to her taskmaster: duty. It seemed like her body and soul were rebalancing a lifetime of sleep deficit. Although I wanted to stroke Mom's head and hold her hand, the hospice nurses discouraged me from doing so. "Death is a private affair not to be shared with anyone but the individuals themselves." Therefore, I sat in a chair by her bed, read the Bible, and prayed my prayer over her, giving her the space to experience one of life's most sacrosanct moments. Believing she could still hear me, I told her that it was okay for her to leave and that we would all be fine like a husband encouraging and coaching his wife during labor.

AN EXHALE

It was now day five of my bedside vigil with Mom. The next day, Sunday, February 12, began day six. Mom panted like a woman in labor straining to give birth. Mom, however, was birthing her own soul into another realm. Her body and feet, now purple, evidenced death's proximity. My husband called to tell me he would pick me up to attend church located next door to the memory-care center. The next morning I met him out front. I really didn't want to go but had not spent any time with him in the past five days. The sermon became background noise as I questioned myself: Why was I there "attending" church when I should have been next door "being" the church? The thought overtook me, and a desperate unction came over my spirit that I had to get back to Mom immediately.

"Take me back right away."

My husband dropped me off at the front door. I rushed through the main entrance, ran down the ninety-foot-long hallway, pushed my way through the coded doors, ran to Mom's room, flung open the door, and exhaled. Mom was still panting. She was still alive. I thanked God for answering my prayer to be with her when she died. Family, being the most important part of her life, was whom she would have wanted by her side. I also believe that, if possible, no one should experience sacred moments such as birth and death alone. My desire was for her, as she left her body, to see family, to see me, someone who loved, honored, and valued her role in my life enough to be present. There was nothing else more important than being by her side.

I sat next to her bed, laid my hands on her head, and prayed my prayer. Mom remained motionless as she had for the past few days. I then read her the Bible and prayed some more. I did not know what else to do but just be there as she would have desired. It had been ten minutes since my arrival. As I sat next to her, feeling how tired I was from not having slept for the last five nights, suddenly

Mom's right shoulder lunged toward me two times as if someone were behind her, pushing her body forward. "Mom! Mom!"

She released her last breath. Mom had entered heaven's gate and was now reborn standing at the threshold of eternity, healed and whole. I sat in silence amazed that the crescendo of our exhausting and complicated journey ended with a simple exhale.

Unlike most mothers who witness their children's first breaths, and motherhood begins, I experienced my mother-child's last breath, and my role as mother ended. She was there to greet me into this world. I was there to say good-bye as she exited this world. A mother's love embraces her newborn with tears of joy. My love released her into the new journey that awaited her because life is changed; it is not taken away. This is the victory of my faith.

In the quiet of my heart, I celebrated the freedom she was now experiencing from the bondage of her body. My emotions, like a wet rag completely wrung out, were void of tears, having mourned every stage of loss over the past eight years. I had made it to the finish line, and I was empty.

I called my brother countless times, but he was attending church and did not answer. I could not comprehend that his cell phone was not with him on vibrate, knowing Mom was so near death. Moreover, I could not fathom why he would not have wanted to be by her side. How I wished he would have wanted to be there that day with me and with her, but in my disappointment I concluded that he did not need as much as I had needed from her; he had gotten it all a long time ago.

REFLECTIONS

THE ANNALS OF WAR

The following week Mom was laid to rest. After eight years of intense warfare, the onslaught of the enemy ceased, and our prolonged conflict ended. Although he was relentless in attacking every part of my physical, emotional, and mental being, defeating and knocking me down in countless battles, I got up every time. The enemy did not know that this was not my first fight in life's journey. I was a veteran. Recruits may fold, but veterans fight, knowing our lives count for another. This is the heart of a soldier. Even though I was a veteran, I never experienced an emotional "world war," a war where one's world is turned upside down. Now that I have, I can say that it developed me into a more seasoned and tenacious warrior for any future attacks in life. I do not give the enemy any recognition because I know that he was just a pawn in God's sovereign hand.

God promises us that while we are on this earth, adversity will enter into our lives. But He is ever present in our time of need because when we are distressed and afflicted, so is He (John 16:33, Isaiah 63:9). To this I can attest because through my adversity He showed me a dimension of His grace that I had never known. His strength was made perfect in my weakness (II Corinthians 12:9). The enemy did cause a tsunami of emotional pain and adversity in my life, but pain is one of God's currencies. He takes our pain and gives us internal riches that surpass the pain we experienced. Through the enemy's hand, God exposed the undesired contents He found resident in my heart. Only the heat and pain of the crucible could have eradicated such ugliness occupying my soul while deeply purifying and tenderizing my heart. In the end, I realized that God had built in me a stead fast character and taught me patience through the adversity I endured (Romans 5:3-4).

Although God remained silent during my time of testing, He never left me or abandon me, as He promises (Hebrews 13:5). What the enemy intended for harm, God determined for my good. He increased and fortified my faith, so weakened in wartime, by resurrecting our entire situation, thereby nullifying every warring act of the enemy because the love of God is a transforming love.

Without my giving birth, He gave me the experience of motherhood along with a mother's heart. God answered; not the prayer on my lips, to heal Mom's temporal physical health, but instead He answered a prayer deep in my heart that I thought was past fulfillment. He healed our souls – something that would never die. The healing I expected and the healing we received made me stand in gratitude and awe of God. His ways are truly higher than our ways, His thoughts higher than our thoughts, and His answers better than our limited requests. He prepared Mom for her next journey and me for the balance of my life. He gave me the mother I always longed for and Mom the daughter she had always desired. He gave us the opportunity to discover that we did like one another, and we became best friends. He turned my tears of pain into joy and laughter. He healed our broken hearts and taught us that on the other side of intimacy is true love. He showed me that the love that grew between us was my true inheritance. However, most importantly, God gave me a revelation of the love weaponry inside my heart as the means to win any future battle because sacrificial love always leads to victory. These were the spoils of my war.

I began this battle from a weak and defensive position. I was defeated along the way, knocked down, and made to cry more than I ever thought I would in my lifetime, but it is not how you start; it is how you finish. It's true that adversity will never leave you where it finds you, but you have a say in where it leaves you.

This fate rests in having a loving and believing attitude toward God even in the face of unanswered questions. When my attitude needed adjusting God loved me to that place of correction. God honors attitude. When it's right towards Him, He manifests Himself. "Blessed are the pure in heart: for they will see God" (Matthew 5:8 NIV). In The Message Bible, the same verse reads, "You're blessed when you get your inside world — your mind and heart — put right. Then you can see God in the outside world."

Early in Mom's illness, I was cautious not to be offended by God or blame Him or put Him on trial and find Him guilty in the courtroom of my mind. I was living between two realities. The natural reality in front of me and the spiritual reality I was expecting to see manifest through my faith. Therefore, with intention, I submitted myself to God's sovereignty and continued believing that I would see a resurrection. I wish I could say that I didn't struggle to keep my mind renewed to God's promises when they didn't manifest according to my timetable. However, what I can say is that I quickly corrected my thinking whenever it faltered. It was a daily walk and not a perfect one. Nevertheless, whatever the outcome was going to be, He was in control whether I understood it or not. In retrospect, if God chose not to restore the relationship between Mom and me, He still used the situation to refashion my heart and show me a dimension of His love I would have never known. There will always be battles in this lifetime but they are opportunities to grow or for God to train us to be stronger in Him. The enemy might have won many battles over the past eight years, but in the end I won the war. My trial ended in triumph, and God alone is to be exalted for my victory.

THE POWER OF SACRIFICIAL LOVE

God considers the needs of any human being holy because all were created in His image. He loves each person to whom He has given His breath of life. When we love one another, we love Him. We are His servants on earth to see that human needs are met through the power of love, and at times that love is sacrificial.

I remember Mom saying throughout her life that she did not want to be a burden to us in her old age. Over these years I learned that truly loving someone is a burden, not in the sense of a problem but a weight that pulls on your heart. Many believe you are carrying a burden that is not yours, but I have learned that it is yours, because the love connecting you to the other person drives you to do things that no one else understands.

It reminds me of my friend's mother, whose hands, raw from the chemicals she used as a beautician, wanted to knit her son a wool sweater. In spite of the pain and bleeding caused by the wooly yarn, she pressed onward, suffering stitch after stitch. Although my friend is a lover of style and clothes, his request is to be buried in that sweater because her sacrifice pierced his heart like nothing else. At his funeral, everyone will wonder why this slave to fashion wanted to be buried in an old, handmade, outdated sweater. The story of her passionate love will be told and her sacrifice memorialized. This love is sacrificial, the highest form of love, a love that compels you to do things no one else can comprehend in spite of pain or loss on your part. No price is too great for the one who becomes a living sacrifice for another. It is the hallmark of true love and its value unsearchable.

My understanding of sacrificial love came into sharp focus during one of our marriage counseling sessions. Addressing his comment toward me, the therapist said, "You need to focus on balancing your emotions about caring for your Mom and caring for yourself."

Oh, is that what I need to do? my mind retorted. He made it sound so easy. Did he not think I had already tried that countless times? I was tired of hearing textbook answers, void of experience, while he believed he reached into the complexities of my heart with a solution. I had no vocabulary to convey the ardor of my emotional roots being ripped out or my daily struggle in managing my heart, wrestling between pain and passion. I realized that in the realm of true love, pain and passion exist together, sharing the same DNA like Siamese twins. When you see one, you see the other. They are inseparable. When you feel pain, you feel passion, and when you feel passion, you feel pain. His well-intended yet buttoned-up advice told me he did not understand that passionate love knows no boundaries or balance. Moreover, it is, at times irrational, reckless, unpredictable, extreme, and, more times than not, sacrificial. He would not have understood that passionate love held me in bondage, but to its shackles I willingly offered my wrists. He would not have understood that God was using the pain of love's bondage to enlarge my heart. When this process was complete then emancipation would be granted. I wished I could get him to understand experientially the words lived out by Mother Teresa: "You love until there is pain; you love through the pain until all that remains is love." He didn't understand that it was necessary for me to drink this cup of suffering, but when you suffer for love's sake, it leads to unspeakable joy. Therefore, I just shook my head in agreement.

This was not the first time I heard this well-intended advice. People continually cautioned me to care for myself while caring for Mom. Although I appreciated their practical wisdom and intentions, they did not understand that while tending to Mom's needs, I met my own. When she hurt, I hurt. When I made her comfortable and happy, I reaped the same. Throughout my life I thought my struggle for independence hinged on discovering where Mom ended and I began. Only after this journey did I realize that there was no delineation. I no longer needed or wanted to be independent from her. Love had melded us into one and became the pure, absolute, and invisible thread that knitted our hearts together. This is love's bond of perfection and ultimate end.

Mom made a difference in my life, and I wanted to make a difference in hers. Sacrificial love was the channel that allowed me to make that difference. Little did I know that my desire would get me drafted into love's boot camp. In retrospect I wished I could have loved more fully, recalling the many times when I fell short because the best and worst came out of me on the battlefield. When my worst came out, love does what love is—it exposed my lack of patience, gentleness, kindness, respect, self-control, or graciousness. Love waits patiently for you to agree with its judgment, plead guilty for not loving, and submit to its ways. Love's work is to prune the unloving tendencies out of our souls so that we can become like a fruit bearing tree. When I did submit to its ways, love set me free by enlarging my heart until my next failure to love. In the domain of love, we are all unfinished works in progress. I learned that when I willingly sacrificed my life for Mom, in spite of the pain, my heart was transformed. Yes, my entire life revolved around Mom, but by the end of that journey, my love life evolved because of her.

SERVANTHOOD

The twelve apostles asked Jesus who would be the greatest in heaven. One would expect a highly structured and magnanimous answer from the Rabbi to define what greatness looks like in the eyes of God. However, Jesus's response was not laced with grandeur but unadorned humility. "The greatest among you will be your servant" (Matthew 23:11 NIV). Service is love in its purist form. Mom always thought of herself as the least; however, in God's eyes, He counted her as one of His greatest. Even though Mom was ill, she continued to serve and be vital to those around her in spite of the enemy's attempts.

Because Mom loved to serve and served to love others, she always recognized and valued servants. One day she displayed her appreciation with unabashed intimacy. Whenever we drove, I always held her hand in between shifting gears. One day she took my right hand in both her hands. With her eyes closed, she kissed my palm as she did from time to time while sitting on the couch. However, this day, she slowly and methodically continued kissing the palm of my hand then proceeded to the reverse side of my hand, every finger, front and back, for about fifteen minutes, forcing me to steer and shift with my left hand. I said nothing, and she said nothing because true intimacy is love's zenith, existing in a realm where words are extraneous, unwelcomed, and dispensable. I never had such a moving and intimate experience. Kissing my hand was her way of honoring another servant. Having been a quintessential servant herself made her most appreciative of the service she had been receiving for the first time in her life. Servanthood was the currency she invested into her family and the dividend she received. It is her legacy that echoes beyond the grave.

There is no question that my marriage suffered damage during Mom's illness. However, after experiencing the "for better or worse" of our wedding vows, we grew to a greater understanding of each other. It is easy serving our spouses during "the better" seasons. However, serving them in "the worse" seasons is difficult because emotions are sometimes raw, angry, or exhausted. The ugliness of our fallen humanity challenged our wedding vows requiring forgiveness on both our parts. We learned that forgiveness is not an event. It is a process. Over time, our mutual forgiveness not only healed our marriage, but also made it stronger.

2013—ONE YEAR LATER

WOMAN IN THE CARD STORE

It was 2013; Mom was born into her new life a year earlier. In my continuing saga to regain my health, I drove from New Jersey to an acupuncturist in Philadelphia that I had gone to in years past. As I drove, I wondered if she would remember me. That particular day was community acupuncture, meaning that the practitioner treats everyone in the same room. Whispering was the protocol to maintain privacy and the peace-filled atmosphere. I sat in the reclining chair as the soft music waltzed its way around the dimly lit room. Lauren sat on a short stool next to my reclining chair. I envied her countenance glowing with health.

She smiled and said, "Hi! It's nice to see you. How are you? I have not seen you in a long time."

"I didn't think you'd remember me."

"I do. What's been going on? What can I do for you?"

"Well, I haven't been here for so long because I've been taking care of my mom, who died a year ago of Alzheimer's disease, and my health took a hit. I'm here for a diagnosis and for you to rebalance and support my energies during my healing process."

Her beautiful smile became somber, conveying deep compassion.

"I'm sorry. I have many female clients who are going through the same thing. It must have been very difficult. How are you doing?"

Like Tracey, Mom's hospice-care nurse, a smile beamed across over my face.

"It was actually the most difficult thing I've ever had to do and the most beautiful experience I've ever had. The disease broke Mom open like a perfume bottle, and the fragrance of love poured out and healed our relationship. If I had to do it all over, I would do it in a heartbeat. It was also the hardest thing I've ever done, but it was the most fun I ever had doing the hardest thing."

With a stunned look, Lauren let her smile return.

"That's such a beautiful picture. I never heard anyone say that before."

After she took my pulses and inserted the needles, I reclined back and closed my eyes for the next hour.

Immediately, my mind flashed back to the woman in the Houston card store years earlier whose voice the enemy had silenced in defeat. She had become a casualty in her war. I wished I could meet her again to tell her that my test had become my testimony and my caretaking experience a sacred privilege. The invisible baton that she silently passed me years earlier I carried over the finish line—exhausted but nonetheless victorious. I now pass you the baton and hope that you, too, will count the spoils of your war and would commit to do it over again.

Loving sacrificially is very expensive because it will always cost you something, and at times it will cost you everything. It is among the highest of callings and the steepest of climbs. If you submit to its call, you will not only reach its summit, but your heart will also reach a new pinnacle and awaken something within you and your loved one.

My prayer is that God give you a revelation of His love that awakens you to a revolution of His love so you can see a resurrection of His love amid your situation.

I encourage you to put on your love weaponry for whatever caretaking challenge awaits you and, with the heart of a soldier, fight your war from a place of sacrificial love and unbridled passions. Doing so will transform your heart and turn your caretaking journey into a pilgrimage.

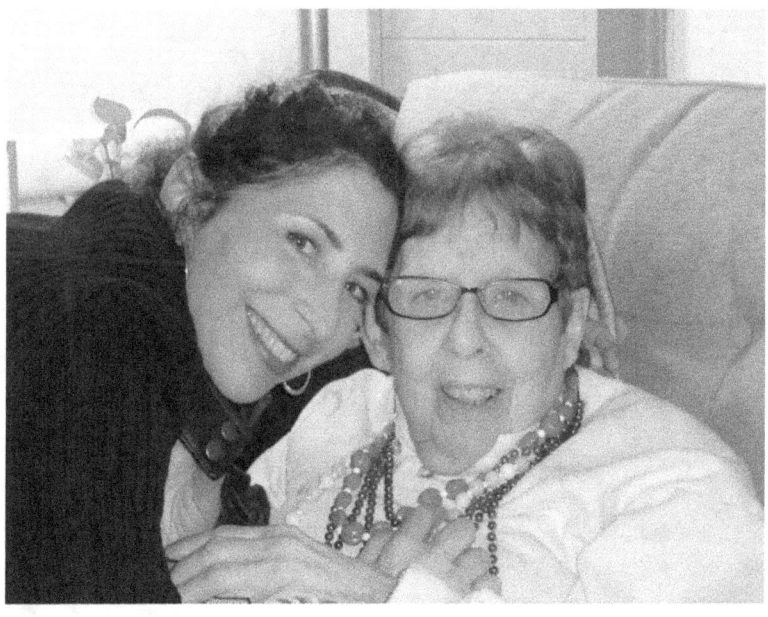

Me and Mom with our hearts knitted together.

Epilogue

All during this journey with Mom, my mind rehearsed the day of her funeral and what I would say for her eulogy. The days prior to her funeral, exhaustion prevented me from writing anything nor did I have the emotional composure to deliver it. My intention was to use Matthew 23:11 as a springboard to tell of Mom's servanthood.

After writing this book, I realized that this work was my eulogy. I wrote it from my heart, hoping to honor her contribution to those whom her life touched. The core of her essence was servanthood. It was the highest expression of her love and the highest expression of love for anyone who serves.

NOTES

MAY 25, 2010–DECEMBER 31, 2010
SURRENDERING TERRITORY
Dear Reader,
Below is the prayer my brother and I said daily over Mom.
By replacing your loved one's name in the appropriate
places, you can make this prayer your own.

Father,
You tell us in Psalm 37:4 to delight ourselves in the Lord
and He will give us the desires of our hearts.

Our desire in writing this petition is to declare Your Word
over Mom, and because it is Your Word, we know it is
Your will for her. You say in Matthew 18:19 that if two of
you shall agree on earth as touching anything that they
shall ask, it shall be done for them of my Father, which is
in heaven. We agree and declare by faith that You did not
give Mom a spirit of fear but of power and of love and of
a sound mind (II Timothy. 1:7). This is our foundational
scripture.

You tell us, Lord, that we wrestle not against flesh and
blood but against principalities, against powers, against
the rulers of the darkness of this world, against spiritual

wickedness in high places. Therefore, we take the whole Armor of God standing with our loins girt about with the truth of Your word; having on the breastplate of righteousness given to us by Jesus, we take the sword of faith to quench the fiery darts of the wicked. We wear the helmet of salvation, thinking with a renewed mind and the sword of the Spirit, which is the Word of God (Ephesians.6:12-17). For we know that the Word of God is quick and powerful and sharper than any two-edged sword (Hebrews 4:12). With this Armor, we take authority over the devil and his stronghold over Mom's mind and health. We bind him according to Matthew 16:19, which states that You will give us the keys of the kingdom of heaven, and whatsoever we shall bind on earth shall be bound in heaven, and whatsoever we shall loose on earth shall be loosed in heaven. We loose from heaven a sound mind, a mind void of confusion because we know that you are not the Author of confusion and disorder but of peace and order (I Corinthians 14:33). We bind all the amyloid protein and plaque in her brain and we command every brain cell to be restored. We plead the blood of Jesus over all of Mom's cells and memories and we call forth full restoration of her brain.

You tell us you are the Lord that heals us (Exodus 15:26). We call on you as Jehovah Rapha, the Lord, our healer, Who His own self bore our sins in His own body on the tree that we, being dead to sins, should live unto righteousness: by whose stripes you were healed (I Peter 2:24). We stand in the gap for our mom as intercessors and ask for forgiveness for her sins (Ezekiel 22:30). We are asking for total healing of our mother's wounded soul and body because You said to your daughter Corinne,

"Beloved I wish above all things that thou may prosper and be in health, even as thy soul prospers" (III John 2). We know that, Jesus, You are King of Kings and Lord of Lords and that God highly exalted You and gave You a name that is above every name. Your name is above the name of any disease, even Alzheimer's (Revelation 19:16, Philippians 2:9).

By faith, we know that you already healed her of all sickness and disease, and we remind you of Nahum 1:9 that this affliction shall not rise up a second time. We give you the praise, God, that our mother honored her father and mother, as the Lord thy God hath commanded; that her days may be prolonged and that it may go well with her in the land which the Lord thy God giveth thee (Deuteronomy 5:16).

We see throughout Your Word that we are our own prophets by the power of our confession. That we shall decree a thing, and it shall be established unto thee, and the light shall shine upon thy ways (Job 22:28).

We believe that this petition has the attention of heaven and that we will have the desires of our hearts for Mom to have a sound mind void of confusion because Jesus came that she might have life and have it more abundantly (John 10:10). This is the confidence that we have in You, that if we ask anything according to Your Will that You hear us: and if we know that You hear us whatsoever we ask, we know that we have the petitions that we desire of You (I John 5:14-15). And we pray this in the mighty name of Jesus. Amen.